THE HERBAL APOTHECARY HANDBOOK

260 Simple Home Remedies for Common Ailments, Plant-powered Wellness, and Natural Self Care

JAMES J CORK

TABLE OF CONTENTS

PART THREE: SAFE AND PRACTICAL PRACTICES

PART ONE:

FOUNDATIONS OF THE MODERN HERBAL APOTHECARY

INTRODUCTION

Did you know that in ancient Egypt, garlic was so prized for its health benefits that it was used as currency to pay the workers who built the pyramids? They believed it boosted strength and endurance – turns out the ancient Egyptians were onto something, because modern research suggests that garlic can enhance immune function and reduce fatigue (Arreola et al., 2015). Who knew this pungent little culinary herb packed such a powerful punch? But garlic is not the only powerful little plant. Nature is the original pharmacy, and our ancestors relied on it extensively.

From the wisdom of herbalists to the age-old practices of indigenous cultures, herbal medicine invites us to connect with nature in a way that many have lost in today's fast-paced world. But why should we care? What could the art of herbalism offer us now, in an era dominated by synthetic drugs and technology? A lot, actually!

Herbal medicine is more than a collection of remedies; it's a transformative experience – one that connects us deeply with our environment, encourages mindfulness, and empowers us towards self-sufficiency. I had a few positive experiences with herbal remedies growing up. My parents loved gardening, and although they weren't herbalists they knew a lot about plants and often had useful tips. When I struggled to sleep, my mom would tuck a sprig of lavender under my pillow. My dad, who had been a Boy Scout leader, knew to rub soft heather fronds on ant bites to soothe the sting. During my teenage years, I dealt with terrible acne, and one of my mom's friends suggested trying nettle tea. It seemed a bit strange, and it tasted funny too, but the results were good enough that I brewed it regularly.

These experiences sparked a deep fascination and respect for nature's pharmacy and its incredible ability to heal in sometimes unexpected ways. I firmly believe that the healing gifts of nature should be accessible to everyone, and that's where this book comes in. Each chapter is designed to guide you on your journey into herbal medicine, whether you're a curious beginner or a seasoned herbalist. There's something in this guide for everyone. In the chapters that follow, you'll discover:

- The foundations of herbal medicine, the tools you'll need, and how to source quality herbal materials.
- A mini compendium of useful herbs for easy reference, so you can quickly look up any herbs whenever you're unsure or need guidance.
- Practical remedies to treat a variety of common conditions.
- Safety and dosage guidelines, and much more.

This book is an invitation to rethink wellness. As we explore the wonders of nature's plant-powered pharmacy together, I encourage you to open your mind and your senses. Feel the textures, inhale the aromas, and taste the vitality that herbal medicine offers. Let every chapter be a step deeper into a world where healing grows quietly and persistently at our feet, waiting patiently to change the way we live, one leaf at a time.

CHAPTER 1:

THE POWER OF A HOME APOTHECARY

The goal of life is living in agreement with nature. –Zeno

Creating a herbal home apothecary is a way of embracing the natural gifts that are abundant in the world around us. It's an open invitation to explore personal solutions to everyday ailments that are as simple as they are natural. The art of cultivating these remedies not only offers us a glimpse into the past, rekindling a connection to traditional practices, but it is also an opportunity to address health concerns with a gentle touch. In this chapter, we'll take a look at the benefits of having a home apothecary, as well as ways to make this practice a sustainable part of our daily routines. Let's get started!

WHY A HOME APOTHECARY? THE BENEFITS OF NATURAL HEALING

Around 40% of today's pharmaceutical products are based on natural ingredients, with many landmark drugs inspired by traditional medicine (Traditional Medicine, 2023). So, having an apothecary in your home just makes sense from both a medical and practical viewpoint. Apart from saving on fuel (because you won't need to rush to the pharmacy for every minor ailment), the practice roots itself in traditions that have been nurtured over generations, empowering us to take control of our health by putting the healing power back in our hands.

One of the biggest benefits of having a home apothecary at your disposal is the sense of independence that comes with it. By cultivating a deeper knowledge of natural remedies, you can attend to everyday health issues using ingredients often found right at home. This not only deepens our connection with nature, but also encourages a deeper understanding of our bodies and how they react to different treatments.

Beyond empowerment, a home apothecary gives us more control over what enters our bodies. Synthetic chemicals in many over-the-counter medicines come with side effects and potential risks that natural alternatives might avoid (Lieberman, 2023).

Did I mention that having a well-stocked and maintained home apothecary can be incredibly budget-friendly? Purchasing medications frequently adds up, especially when dealing with chronic conditions. In contrast, natural remedies often involve affordable, readily available ingredients. Growing herbs at home, such as peppermint or thyme, can give us an ongoing supply of medicinal plants that can be harvested as needed. Cultivating your own plants requires minimal resources and helps conserve biodiversity, so that's a win for nature as well as your wallet (White, 2019).

As an added bonus, creating your own herbal medicines almost demands that we become more mindful in our everyday lives. Making your own remedies is a great way to slow down and connect with nature. Taking care of plants and using them thoughtfully brings a sense of calm and helps cut through the chaos of daily life. It also preserves ancient traditions, reminding us of how closely we are linked to the environment. It's a practice that's both beautiful and easy to get started.

STARTING ESSENTIALS

Plastic is the enemy in any apothecary. There are two main reasons to avoid using plastics for herbal preparations. First, plastics can leach unwanted chemicals into our remedies, which may be harmful to our cells (Zimmermann et al., 2021). Second, plastics degrade in a unique way. Unlike natural materials like wood, which eventually break down into their basic elements, plastics degrade into tiny, uneven pieces called microplastics. These microplastics can enter our bloodstream, accumulate in our bodies, and potentially cause various health problems (Leslie et al., 2022). So, a golden rule any practicing and aspiring herbalist should follow is to banish plastics in all their incarnations from the apothecary. Some of the essential tools you'll need may include:

- **Mortar and pestle:** A quality mortar and pestle are indispensable companions in grinding herbs into fine powders or making pastes. This ancient tool offers a tactile connection to the practices of our ancestors, blending ingredients manually – a satisfying ritual that also helps preserve the integrity of delicate herb components. Use a stainless steel one where possible, as they are durable, easy to clean, and suitable for both soft and woody herbal material. Granite is another good option, as they do not absorb oils or flavors and can be used to grind herbal materials into fine powders. Avoid wood as it will absorb oils and flavors, making them a nightmare to clean, which can impact the integrity of our herbal preparations.
- **Glass jars:** For all your storage needs, turn to glass. They are non-reactive and help protect contents from moisture and air exposure, maintaining freshness and potency.
- **Muslin cloths:** Versatile and useful for straining infused oils or crafting herbal sachets. Always opt for unbleached muslin cloth

wherever possible, as bleached cloth may leave behind trace chemicals in our preparations.

These tools form the backbone of an effective apothecary, facilitating the preparation and organization of remedies. But we've only scratched the surface here. Head to Chapter Two for a detailed exploration of all the tools you'll need to get started.

Arrange your space to ensure your collection is accessible and inviting. For those starting this journey, begin with familiar favorites – perhaps five or ten most-used herbs – and gradually expand as your knowledge grows. Embrace this process as ongoing rather than static, shaping your apothecary according to evolving needs and preferences.

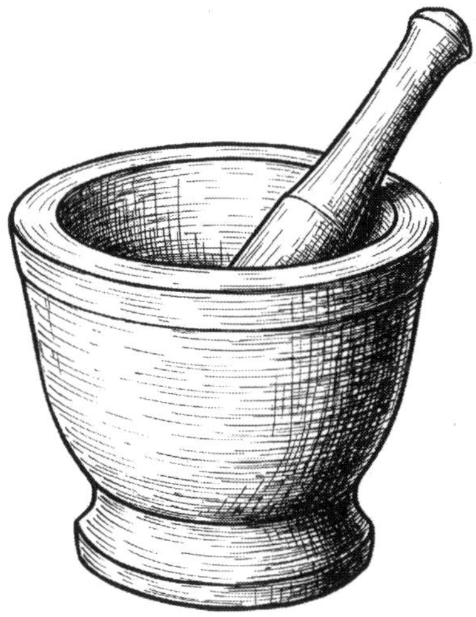

THE MOST VERSATILE REMEDIES YOU CAN START USING TODAY

Versatile remedies you can stock your apothecary with include simple salves, teas, and pantry-based remedies. The following remedies will give you a solid foundation for your apothecary that you can build on:

Remedy	Type and uses
Healing salves	Calendula, comfrey and beeswax-based salves can be used to treat skin wounds, insect bites, and stings (Saras, 2025).
Herbal teas and infusions	Chamomile tea to promote peaceful sleep and peppermint tea to aid digestion (Boling, 2010).
Pantry-based cures	Honey can be used to soothe sore throats, whilst apple cider vinegar can be useful to boost immunity (Saras, 2025).

THE ROOTS OF THE HOME APOTHECARY: A BRIEF HISTORY

To truly appreciate the power of a home apothecary, it helps to understand its origins. For centuries, apothecaries were at the heart of community health, blending the art of herbal medicine with a deep knowledge of natural remedies. These practices not only laid the groundwork for modern pharmacies but also offer timeless wisdom that's making a comeback today.

ANCIENT HEALING TRADITIONS

The origins of home apothecaries trace back thousands of years to ancient civilizations such as Egypt, China, India (through Ayurveda), and Greece. In ancient Egypt, healers utilized a variety of herbs, resins, and oils for medicinal purposes, as documented in texts like the Ebers Papyrus, which dates to around 1550 BCE. Similarly, traditional Chinese medicine incorporated complex herbal formulations, many of which remain in use today. In India, the Ayurvedic system emphasized balancing bodily energies through the use of herbs and spices, a practice that continues to influence modern holistic approaches. Greek scholars, including Hippocrates and Dioscorides, cataloged numerous medicinal plants, laying the foundation for Western herbalism (Pan et al., 2014). These traditions share a common belief that nature offers remedies essential for human health.

MEDIEVAL AND COLONIAL APOTHECARIES

In medieval Europe, apothecaries were essential healthcare providers, offering medicinal herbs, spices, and general medical advice. Their shops were often filled with a variety of concoctions, such as "oil of swallows" and "syrup of serpents," reflecting the medical practices of the time.

In colonial America, apothecaries continued this tradition, serving as both pharmacists and general practitioners. They prepared and dispensed medicines, diagnosed illnesses, and provided treatments using locally sourced plants. Their shops were stocked with dried herbs, tinctures, and salves, stored in glass jars and wooden drawers, embodying a blend of folk wisdom and emerging scientific practices (Gill, 1972).

WHY THEY DISAPPEARED

Over time, the roles of apothecaries evolved, leading to the specialized fields of pharmacy and medicine we recognize today. However, the foundational practices of apothecaries have experienced a resurgence, with modern home apothecaries drawing inspiration from these historical traditions to promote natural and holistic approaches to health (Wust, 2017).

INTEGRATING APOTHECARY PRACTICES INTO DAILY LIFE

Contrary to popular belief, making natural remedies a part of your daily life does not have to be a complicated affair. In fact, it can be very rewarding and empowering. Herbal infusions are excellent natural alternatives to over-the-counter medications, often used for common ailments. For centuries, cultures worldwide have turned to the calming properties of chamomile tea to aid in a restful night's sleep (Hassen et al., 2022).

Transitioning from commercial skincare and beauty products to natural skincare is another effortless way we can make nature a part of our daily routine. Our skin tends to absorb everything we apply to it, and it's the largest organ. This makes it crucial to scrutinize product ingredients. Natural alternatives like aloe vera, coconut oil, and honey help hydrate and rejuvenate the skin without harmful chemicals (Shenefelt, 2011). Creating DIY facial masks or body scrubs using these natural ingredients not only ensures you're nurturing your skin with safe and effective remedies, but it's also a fun bit of self-care.

Another essential aspect of a home apothecary is maintaining a quick-access remedy kit. This kit acts as your first line of defense in emergencies, offering ready-made natural solutions for minor injuries or common ailments. Simple ingredients like activated charcoal for upset stomachs or lavender oil for minor cuts transform an ordinary cabinet into a powerful healing station.

The simplicity of apothecary practices is what allowed a busy mother of four to take care of her children's health naturally. By keeping simple, natural remedies on hand, she's able to treat fevers, minor cuts, sinus problems, stomach issues, pain, and bleeding whenever they arise without needing to rush to the pharmacy (Dietrich-Marsh, 2020). This transition to natural alternatives was not; instead, it was a gradual replacement strategy that involved research, careful selection of herbs and remedies, and commitment to understanding their benefits. Over time, she saw improvements in immunity, energy levels, and general health in her children.

While these practices hold great promise, it's crucial to approach them with informed caution. Herbal supplements, despite their natural origin, present risks when misused or when interactions are overlooked (Hassen et al., 2022). But we'll discuss this in more detail in Part Three. The knowledge shared in that section aims to empower you to use natural remedies effectively and safely.

Embracing the time-honored wisdom of herbal remedies not only frees us from a full reliance on commercial pharmaceuticals but also deepens our connection to our bodies and the natural world. In the next chapter, we'll thoroughly explore all the essentials needed to get your home apothecary started.

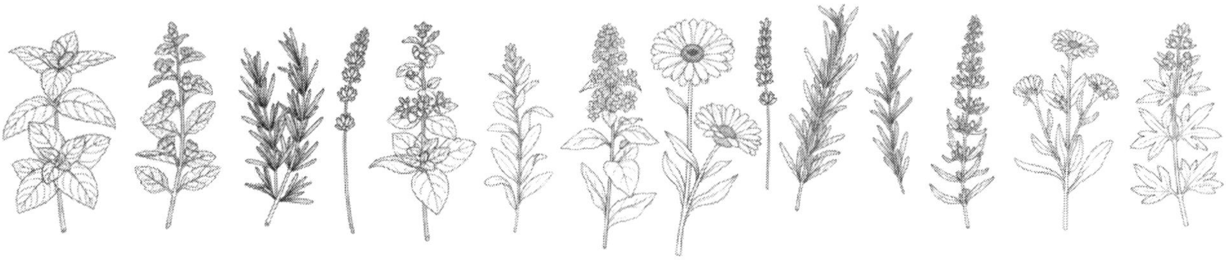

CHAPTER 2:

TOOLS AND INGREDIENTS YOU NEED

I firmly believe that nature brings solace in all troubles. –Anne Frank

Building an efficient apothecary involves more than just gathering herbs; it's about having the right equipment and understanding how each tool contributes to the process.

In the previous chapter, we've touched on some of the tools needed, but in this chapter, you'll find a detailed explanation of all the essentials you will need to make homemade herbal remedies of the highest quality. Additionally, you'll learn about the core ingredients that lay the foundation for many natural treatments, from versatile dried herbs to diverse solvents that extract their therapeutic properties.

ESSENTIAL TOOLS AND STORAGE SOLUTIONS FOR YOUR HOME APOTHECARY

In Chapter One, I mentioned that essentials like the mortar and pestle, glass jars, and muslin clothes make up the basic toolkit for your home apothecary. However, there are still a couple of important points to cover. While granite or stainless steel pestles and mortars are excellent choices, it's crucial to keep your apothecary tools separate from your kitchen ones. Using the same mortar and pestle for both can compromise the quality of your herbal remedies. Your mortar and pestle should be dedicated exclusively to your apothecary work to ensure the purity and effectiveness of your creations.

A spice grinder can be used, but there are a few things to keep in mind. Spice grinders are great for quickly grinding herbs and spices, especially if you're working with larger quantities or need a finer consistency. However, they may not preserve the integrity of delicate plant compounds. On top of this, there is a risk of cross-contaminating your herbal remedies with leftover spices or other substances. Whether you use a spice grinder or a mortar and pestle, the key is to ensure that you're maintaining the purity of your herbs by keeping the tools clean.

Sterilizing glass jars before storing anything in them is always a good idea. Wash the jar in hot, soapy water and give it a thorough rinse.. While the jar is still damp, microwave it on high for one to two minutes to help kill any lingering bacteria. Remember: No metal objects in the microwave, and give the jar plenty of time to cool down before using. Taking this simple step has saved a lot of my herbal remedies from going rancid!

Wherever possible, use amber vessels to store light-sensitive remedies. Amber colored glass is known to block light, which can help to extend the shelf life of tinctures and oils. Mason jars are great to store larger quantities of dried herbs, but reserve your amber bottles for liquid extracts. Ensure your glass jars have airtight seals to prevent contamination. This helps to preserve the potency of your preparations as well.

Equally important is having a reliable set of measuring equipment. Just like with the mortar and pestle, it's best to keep your measuring equipment separate from the kitchen to avoid cross-contamination.

Next, we come to the double boiler, an indispensable tool for the gentle heating of ingredients. Direct heat can destroy valuable medicinal properties or even alter the chemical structure of certain compounds, which can reduce their therapeutic effects. A double boiler setup provides a buffer between your ingredients and the heat source, allowing you to carefully control the temperature and preserve the integrity of your remedies (Calhoun, 2024).

Last but definitely not least, keep labels and a marker on hand. Label your jars with the contents and the date – they'll save you from the classic sniff-and-guess test later on!

FUNDAMENTAL INGREDIENTS AND SAFETY EQUIPMENT

Dried herbs and solvents form the backbone of many natural remedies, so it's a good idea to stock up on staples like chamomile, peppermint, and elderberries. For more information and handy herbs to stock up on, head to Chapter Five.

Then you'll need solvents such as alcohol, apple cider vinegar, or glycerin to turn these herbs into tinctures and salves. These liquids act as carriers, drawing out the active compounds in the herb, so it's important to choose the right one for the job. The table opposite should help you decide which solvent works best for different herbal preparations:

Solvent	Best for	Examples of herbs	Notes
Water	Extracting vitamins, minerals, polysaccharides, and mucilage.	Marshmallow root, chamomile, nettle	Use for teas, infusions, and decoctions. Best for fresh or dried herbs.
Ethanol (Alcohol, 40-60%)	Extracting alkaloids, resins, and essential oils; preserving tinctures.	Echinacea, valerian, and hawthorn berries	Vodka or brandy is common. High-proof alcohol (over 60%) can be too strong for some herbs.
Glycerin	Extracting delicate compounds; alcohol-free alternative.	Lavender, lemon balm, elderberries	Ideal for children and those avoiding alcohol; sweeter taste.
Vinegar	Extracting minerals and alkaloids; preserving and enhancing digestion.	Dandelion, nettle, garlic	Apple cider vinegar is popular; use glass containers to avoid corrosion.
Oil (Olive, coconut, etc.)	Extracting fat-soluble compounds for salves and infusions.	Calendula, St. John's wort, arnica	Use low heat for infusions; store in dark, cool places to prevent rancidity.
Honey	Extracting moisture and mild compounds; preserving syrups.	Elderberry, ginger, thyme	Great for cough syrups and oxymels; avoid for infants under one year due to botulism risk.
Witch hazel (Distillate)	Extracting tannins and astringent compounds for topical use.	Witch hazel bark, calendula, rose petals	Ideal for toners, sprays, and compresses, but not for internal use (Easley & Horne, 2016).

Equally important in your apothecary toolkit are waxes. Beeswax, combined with carrier oils like olive, coconut, or jojoba oil, is foundational in making salves and balms. While beeswax is a versatile staple, it's far from the only wax you can use in your herbal creations. For those ready to explore new options, here's a handy table that breaks down which type of wax works best for different situations:

Type of wax	Properties	Best uses in herbal medicine
Beeswax	Natural, antibacterial, and soothing	Balms, salves, lip balms, barrier creams; solidifies oils without being too hard.
Carnauba wax	Plant-based, harder than beeswax, hypoallergenic	Vegan alternatives to beeswax; balms, salves, and lotions that need a firmer texture.
Candelilla wax	Plant-based, smooth texture, melts at lower temperature	Vegan balms, salves, and lip balms; good for softer consistencies.
Soy wax	Plant-based, soft, lower melting point	Creams, softer salves, and massage bars; suitable for vegan formulations.
Rice bran wax	Plant-based, emulsifying properties	Creams and lotions; helps blend oil and water-based ingredients.
Bayberry wax	Plant-based, aromatic, firmer than beeswax	Specialty balms and salves with a natural fragrance.
Sunflower wax	Plant-based, hard, high melting point	Lipsticks, balms, and salves needing a firmer finish.

The process of creating a balm usually involves gently heating the oils with wax until melted, allowing the mixture to cool, and then solidifying into a usable product.

SAFETY FIRST

Safety cannot be overlooked when working with concentrated herbal preparations and heat sources. Protective gear, such as gloves and eyewear, is vital in ensuring our safety. Gloves protect your skin from irritation and absorption of potent substances like essential oils and plant sap (if working with fresh herbs), which can cause skin irritation or allergic reactions if handled directly. Protective eyewear shields your eyes from potential splashes during the mixing process, especially when dealing with volatile solvents and oils that may cause harm upon contact.

Also, there's the matter of safety beyond simple preparation. Whenever we're working with heat, it's a prudent precaution to keep a fire extinguisher nearby. Often, preparing herbal remedies includes heating oils or herbal mixtures, which carry inherent risks. Having a fire extinguisher on hand ensures that, in the unlikely event of a fire, you can quickly respond, keeping yourself and your workspace safe from harm. For a more detailed exploration of safety in the apothecary, go to Part Three.

With the right tools and ingredients, you're now equipped to begin crafting your own remedies. Next, we'll explore sourcing, growing, and preserving herbs to ensure a sustainable supply for your apothecary.

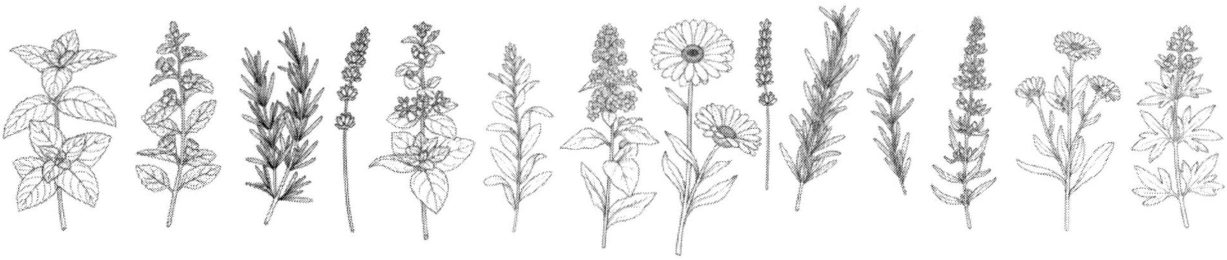

CHAPTER 3:

SOURCING, GROWING AND PRESERVING HERBS

In every walk with nature one receives far more than he seeks. –John Muir

Sourcing, growing, and preserving herbs might sound simple, but it's a vital part of cultivating an effective home apothecary. This chapter invites you into the fascinating world of herbs, guiding you from seed to shelf. We'll explore effective ways to preserve these wonderful green allies, ensuring they retain their maximum potency and healing power.

ETHICAL SOURCING AND CULTIVATION OF HERBS

Relying on nature's gifts means taking on the responsibility of protecting them. When we harvest herbs, we're not just benefiting from what the earth provides – we're also responsible for making sure those resources stay healthy and abundant for the future. Ethically sourcing herbs is about finding that balance between using what we need and giving back to the land that sustains us.

When herbs are ethically sourced, they contribute to environmental sustainability by preserving natural habitats and biodiversity. This ensures that plants continue to grow naturally without being over-harvested or destroyed, which can lead to extinction in some cases. Sadly, this is the case in South Africa and Namibia, where succulent poaching is pushing many species to the brink of extinction (Coleman, 2023). All of this damage is being done to satisfy a selfish market that craves unusual-looking plants. It's a tragedy comparable to Shakespeare's *King Lear*, because once they're lost, no one is able to experience them ever again. This can be done in a few ways:

RESEARCHING OUR SUPPLIERS

Taking the extra steps needed to ensure we are purchasing our herbal supplies from individuals and companies who understand and implement ecological preservation practices. Organic certification is essential, as it guarantees that herbs were grown without harmful pesticides or synthetic fertilizers, while fair trade ensures that the people involved in their production receive fair wages and work under humane conditions.

GROWING YOUR OWN

Growing herbs at home provides an unparalleled level of control over their quality. This not only guarantees freshness and potency but also reduces reliance on external suppliers. The process couldn't be simpler! All you need is some well-drained soil (or a well-draining flower box), plenty of sunlight, and regular watering. However, be careful not to overwater – most herbs prefer soil that's moist but not soggy. Pay attention to each plant's specific needs, and you'll have a thriving herb garden in no time!

PRACTICING SUSTAINABLE WILDCRAFTING

Harvesting wild plants for use requires a deep understanding of local ecosystems. It is about knowing which parts of the plant can be harvested without causing harm, ensuring that the plant can regrow and continue to thrive in its ecosystem. Sustainable wildcrafting respects the cycles of nature, ensuring that plants are picked at the right time and in the right way to promote continual growth and replenishment.

A little more thought and research are required to ensure you're doing it responsibly and sustainably. These tips will help you get started the right way:

- **Know your plants:** Always make sure you can positively identify the plant you're harvesting. Use a reliable field guide or app to avoid any mix-ups with toxic look-alikes.
- **Harvest with care:** Take only what you need. Nothing more. It's essential to leave enough behind for the plant to regenerate and for wildlife to forage. Never harvest an entire plant.
- **Choose abundant species:** Harvesting rare or endangered plants? That's a big no-no. Avoid picking from areas where plants are scarce, ensuring their survival for future generations.
- **Respect local regulations:** Be aware of any local laws or regulations that may govern wildcrafting in your area, especially when it comes to protected species or public land.
- **Minimize your footprint:** Stick to established paths and avoid trampling surrounding plants or disturbing the ecosystem. Take care to leave the environment as you found it.
- **Practice sustainable harvesting:** For perennial plants, consider harvesting only the leaves or flowers rather than uprooting the whole plant. If you're harvesting roots, take only a small portion from mature plants.
- **Know the right time:** Harvesting at the right time ensures the plant's potency and supports its regeneration. Most herbs are best harvested when they are in bloom or during their peak growth season.

By following these tips, you're ensuring that both the plants and the environment thrive for years to come!

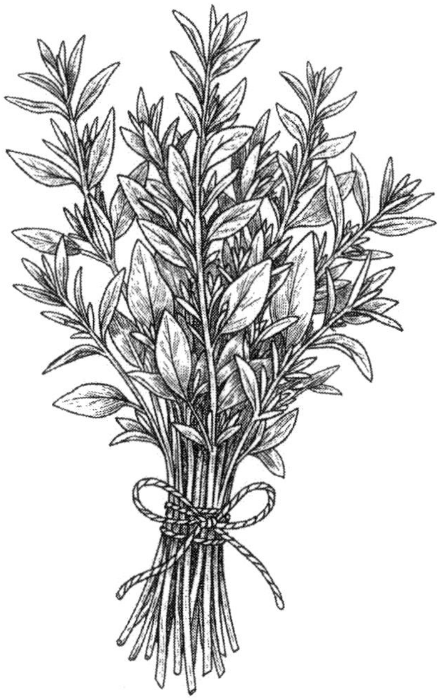

THE BEST HERB HARVESTING AND PRESERVATION STRATEGIES

Now that you've got a sustainable supply of herbs, harvesting and preserving them is vital, so that you can get the highest potency and use them effectively all year round. The essence of herbs lies in their potent oils, which are responsible for much of their medicinal properties. It's important to time your harvest to ensure the maximum concentration of these oils.

The best time to harvest most herbs is in the morning, ideally just after the morning dew has evaporated. This timing ensures that the essential oils have accumulated overnight and are ready for collection. Picking herbs during this period maximizes their efficacy when used in recipes, tinctures, or teas.

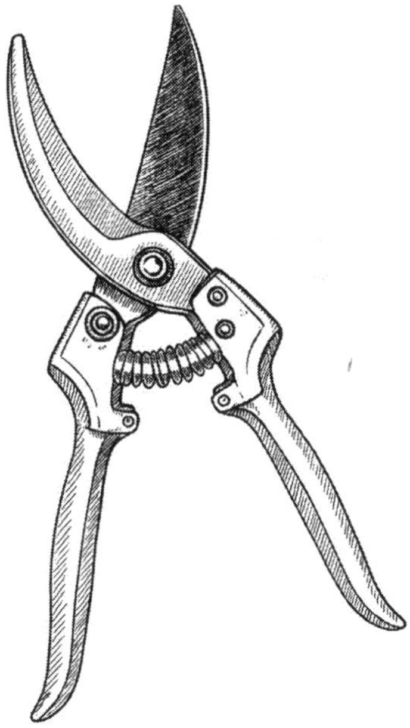

Use sharp pruners or scissors to make clean cuts, reducing damage to the plant. This precise cutting encourages the plant to heal quickly and encourages further growth. Blunt tools can crush stems, leading to potential infections or stunted growth. Properly pruned plants tend to flourish, allowing you to extend your harvesting season.

After careful harvesting, preserving herbs effectively ensures they remain useful throughout the year. Air drying is a traditional method that gently removes moisture while retaining the oils and flavors (Ling, 2024). Common preservation methods include:

Preservation method	Best herbs to use	Details	Tips for best results
Dehydration	Basil, oregano, thyme, rosemary, sage, mint, lemon balm, marjoram	Ideal for woody or semi-woody herbs with low to moderate moisture content. Helps to preserve the flavor and gives the herb a longer shelf life.	Use a dehydrator at 95°F to 115°F. Store in glass jars (airtight) away from sources of heat and light..
Air drying	Lavender, bay leaves, rosemary, sage	Suitable for herbs with sturdy leaves or stems. Involves hanging herbs upside down in a dry, ventilated space.	Bundle stems loosely, tie with twine, and hang in a dark, dry area.
Freezing	Parsley, cilantro, chives, dill, basil, tarragon	Delicate herbs that tend to lose their flavor when dried can be preserved this way. Maintains color and potency.	Chop and freeze in ice cube trays with olive oil or water for easy use in cooking.
Salt preservation	Basil, thyme, rosemary, oregano	Involves layering herbs with salt to draw out moisture while preserving flavor.	Store in airtight containers; use flavored salt directly in recipes.

Consistent harvesting plays a vital role not only in sustaining a fresh supply but also in encouraging regrowth – something this gardener learned through hands-on experience. What began as a small experiment with an oregano plant evolved into a decade-long journey of cultivating a diverse and thriving herb garden. Inspired by the remedies, I learned and the side benefit of using some of these amazing flavors in cooking, my experiment grew from a planter box to a sizable garden bed, with each plant selected for its ability to thrive in the northeastern U.S. climate.

But it wasn't without its challenges! I lost countless plants along the way – sometimes to the elements, sometimes to pests, and other times to my own mistakes (like overwatering). Each loss was a lesson, helping me figure out what truly thrives in my garden. Depending on your location and climate, you may find yourself experimenting as well, learning through trial and error which plants will grow best in your space.

Challenge	The solution
Selecting the right herbs for the climate	Many herbs struggled to survive cold winters, especially more tender varieties. The focus changed to strong plants like oregano, thyme, sage, and chives, which come back every year with little care. Each spring, annuals like basil and cilantro were planted to go along with the perennials.
Harvesting without harming	Over-harvesting left some plants weak and unable to grow back effectively. The key was to harvest small amounts from the plants regularly, but never more than half at once. Plants like mint and parsley were fully cut back in the fall since they die back to the ground naturally. This method helped the plants grow bushier and kept the garden healthy.
Preserving flavor and Potency	Some herbs, such as parsley and cilantro, lose their flavor when dried. Freezing was chosen as the preservation method for delicate herbs, with finely chopped portions stored in labeled freezer bags. Hardier herbs like oregano and thyme were air-dried by bundling them with twine and hanging them in a cool, dark place until crisp, then storing them in glass jars.

By adopting these solutions, the backyard plot was transformed into a reliable source of herbs. The combination of effective harvesting and preservation techniques ensured a continuous supply of herbs throughout the year.

Ethically sourcing, cultivating, and preserving herbs are the cornerstones of ensuring you have a consistent and potent supply for your home apothecary. In the next chapter, we'll explore the preparation of various herbal remedies using these preserved herbs.

CHAPTER 4:

MAKING REMEDIES: TEAS, TINCTURES, AND MORE

Nature does not hurry, yet everything is accomplished. –Lao Tzu

Crafting your own herbal remedies is a powerful way to embrace natural healing and take control of your well-being. In this chapter, we'll explore a variety of preparation methods – from soothing teas and potent tinctures to comforting syrups and healing salves. Along the way, you'll discover practical techniques and tips to help you build a well-rounded and effective home apothecary.

TEAS, INFUSIONS, AND DECOCTIONS

Each extraction method suits different plant components, influencing the versatility and applicability of herbal remedies. Soft, tender leaves are perfect for teas, while hard roots and bark find their strength in decoctions. When in doubt, this handy table can help:

Method	Description	Best herbs for this method	Steeping time	Tips for best results
Tea	A gentle extraction method where herbs are steeped briefly in hot water. Ideal for delicate or aromatic herbs and flowers.	Chamomile, peppermint, lemon balm, lavender, green tea, rooibos, elderflower, lemon verbena	3-10 minutes	Use freshly boiled water, but allow it to cool slightly (about 190°F/88°C) for delicate herbs. Cover the cup to retain heat.
Infusion	A longer steeping method, usually for leaves, flowers, or milder herbs. Offers a more potent extraction than tea.	Nettle, red clover, lemon balm, elderflower, rose, oregano, alfalfa, yarrow	15-30 minutes	Use a heatproof container, steep with a lid to trap essential oils, and steep for a longer period for a stronger flavor.
Decoction	Used for hard, woody, or root herbs that need more intense extraction. The herb is boiled in water and simmered to extract active compounds.	Ginger, dandelion root, licorice root, burdock root, cinnamon bark, turmeric, angelica root	20-45 minutes	Simmer gently on low heat, don't boil aggressively, and strain well. You may need to reduce the liquid slightly for potency.

This gentle process preserves delicate oils and other beneficial compounds, providing both health benefits and a soothing aroma. Brewing and sipping a warm cup of herbal tea offers a calming moment while keeping you hydrated, whether enjoyed alone or with loved ones.

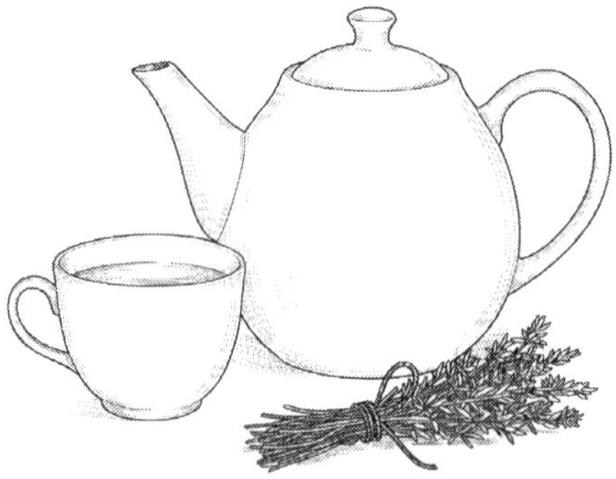

TINCTURES

Tinctures are potent liquid extracts, usually made with alcohol, that capture and concentrate the healing properties of herbs. They offer a powerful way to harness the benefits of plants in a convenient and long-lasting form.

Tincture type	Herbs best suited	Method	Tips for best results
Alcohol tincture (Vodka, brandy, rum)	Echinacea, St. John's wort, lavender, ashwagandha, calendula, oregano, ginger, holy basil	Chop fresh herbs or crush dried herbs. Place herbs in a clean jar, filling it about halfway. Submerge the herbs with alcohol. Seal and shake well. Let it steep in a dark, cool place for 4-6 weeks, shaking daily. Strain and store the liquid in an amber bottle.	Use high-proof alcohol for better extraction. If using fresh herbs, use a 1:2 ratio (one part herbs to two parts alcohol) Ensure herbs are fully submerged to avoid mold.
Glycerite (Vegetable glycerin)	Chamomile, peppermint, lemon balm, raspberry leaf	Follow the same process as for an alcohol tincture. Substitute alcohol with vegetable glycerin. Use a 1:3 ratio of herbs to glycerin. Allow a steeping time of up to four weeks. Agitate the contents daily. Strain and store the contents in an amber bottle.	Glycerin extracts fewer compounds than alcohol, so this method works best with milder herbs. Ideal for children or those avoiding alcohol.

Tincture type	Herbs best suited	Method	Tips for best results
Vinegar tincture (Apple cider vinegar, white vinegar, red wine vinegar, rice vinegar)	Motherwort, ccalendula, garlic, burdock, thyme, rosemary	Prepare herbs as with other tinctures. A ratio of one part herbs to two parts vinegar (1:2) is best. Submerge herbs in vinegar. Seal and store. Allow a steeping time of up to six weeks and agitate the contents daily.. Strain and store in a glass bottle.	Vinegar tinctures provide a more astringent, mineral-rich effect. Apple cider vinegar is most commonly used, but others can impart different flavors or medicinal properties.

To ensure your tincture is still good to use, look for the following signs:

- **Change in smell:** A rancid or sour odor is a clear indication that something has gone wrong. If the smell becomes unpleasant or "off," discard the tincture.
- **Mold or cloudiness:** Mold or excessive cloudiness may form, especially if the herbs weren't fully submerged in the solvent or if the tincture was exposed to air.
- **Separation:** While some separation of herbs and solvent is normal, if the mixture begins to separate significantly, it may be a sign that it's no longer stable.
- **Color:** If the tincture turns an unusual color (like greenish or brownish) after it's been properly stored for a while, it may be starting to degrade.

To prevent tinctures from going bad fast, it's always a good idea to store them in dark glass bottles, in a cool, dry place, and make sure the herbs are fully covered by the solvent.

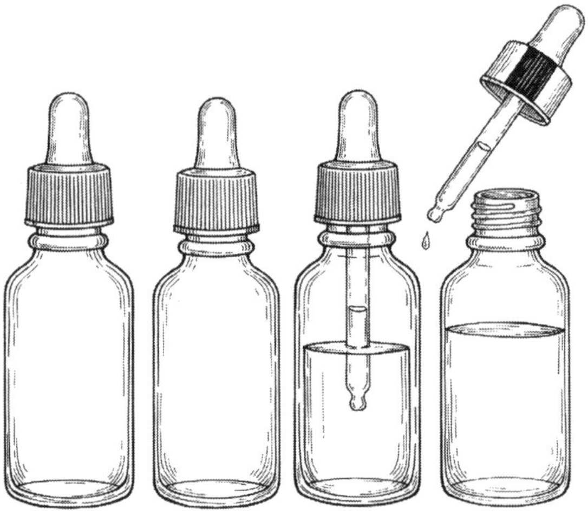

SYRUPS

Herbal syrups are a delightful way to incorporate medicinal herbs into your daily life. These concoctions marry the therapeutic benefits of herbs with the sweetness of honey, maple syrup, or agave, creating a remedy that is not only effective but also appealing to children.

Sweetener	Herbs best suited	Preparation method	Tips for best results
Honey	Elderberry, thyme, chamomile, peppermint, lavender	Make a strong decoction of the desired herbs. Strain the liquid and return it to the pot. Add honey to the decoction, typically in a 1:1 ratio. Warm gently to combine, avoiding boiling.	Use fresh herbs for vibrant flavor. Chamomile and thyme are soothing. Add a small amount of brandy or tincture to extend shelf life. Bottle and store in the refrigerator.
Maple Syrup	Elderberry, ginger, marshmallow root	Same preparation method as with honey-based syrups.	Maple syrup adds a rich flavor, great for elderberry and ginger.
Agave	Lemon balm, licorice root, peppermint	Prepare the same way as honey-based syrups.	Agave's mild sweetness complements minty and licorice flavors.

To ensure your herbal syrups are safe to use, check for signs of spoilage before each use. A syrup that has gone bad may develop mold on the surface, emit an off or fermented smell, or change in color and consistency, becoming unusually cloudy or thicker. Storing syrups in airtight containers in the refrigerator and adding a small amount of alcohol, like brandy, can help extend their shelf life.

SALVES

Salves are a wonderful hands-on way to benefit from the healing properties of herbs by delivering the benefits directly to the skin. Beeswax and oil are the main ingredients you will need. Here's how to turn these simple ingredients into a skin-loving salve:

- Infuse herbs in a carrier oil by heating gently over a double boiler.
- Strain the infused oil to remove plant material.
- Combine the infused oil with beeswax in a ratio of approximately 1 cup of oil to 1 ounce of beeswax. The more beeswax you add to the mixture, the firmer the end product will become.
- Heat until the beeswax melts completely, then pour the liquid into tins or jars and allow to cool and solidify.
- If your salve turns out too soft, you can gently reheat it and stir in some melted beeswax to achieve a firmer texture. On the other hand, if it's too hard, simply reheat the salve and mix in additional infused oil until you reach the desired consistency.

Store the containers away from sources of direct light and heat.. A cupboard or drawer is ideal. Avoid storing salves in the refrigerator unless they contain fresh ingredients that require refrigeration. Salves are simple yet powerful, allowing you to customize them according to your specific skin needs and preferences. Of course, beeswax is not the only type of wax you can use to make salves; see Chapter Two for a detailed list of waxes and their best uses.

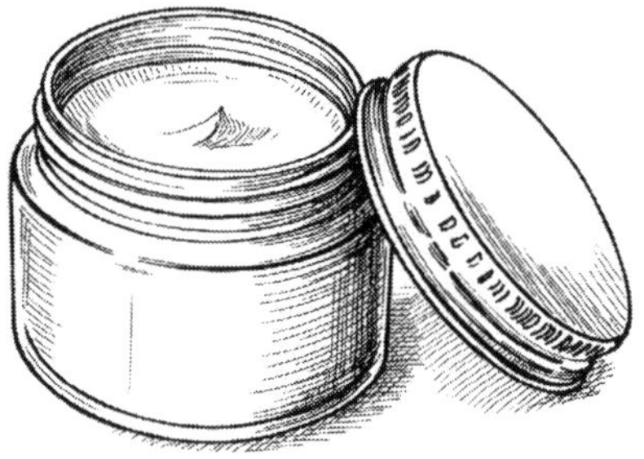

GET HANDS-ON

Exploring herbal remedies is all about getting hands-on and turning theory into practice. Choose one method from above and prepare a remedy using herbs you have sourced or grown. As you go through the process, document any challenges, observations, and adjustments you make along the way. Trying out different methods, making your own remedies, and keeping track of what works can be both fun and enlightening. For beginners, starting with something simple, like a peppermint syrup for digestion or a lavender salve to soothe irritated skin, can help build confidence. As you experiment, jot down notes about what worked, what didn't, and any adjustments you made. This process not only deepens your understanding of herbal preparations but also helps you improve with each attempt.

Learning to craft herbal syrups and salves at home is an empowering way to take control of your health naturally. By understanding how to address common ailments without immediately relying on conventional medicine, you can embrace a more holistic approach to well-being. Additionally, making your own remedies is a sustainable practice that aligns seamlessly with a natural lifestyle. This is precisely what inspired a passionate herbalist whom I know well, who started with a simple exploration into the benefits of chamomile tinctures.

Chamomile is known for its calming effects and ability to promote better sleep. Drawn to its gentle yet effective nature, Carolyn harvested dried chamomile flowers directly from her own herb garden. She decided to create an alcohol-based tincture, selecting 80-proof vodka for its neutral taste and excellent preservative properties. The process came with its challenges. Finding a dark, consistently cool spot for storage was tricky, and it was tempting to strain the tincture too soon. However, patience prevailed, resulting in a powerful and effective remedy. Taking 20–30 drops diluted in warm water about 30 minutes before bedtime made it easier to fall asleep and wake up feeling refreshed (Thomas, 2023). The tincture's calming properties also proved invaluable during stressful days, offering a natural way to unwind without the drowsiness often caused by over-the-counter sleep aids..

Crafting your own herbal remedies is a journey that combines the wisdom of nature with personal empowerment. Mastering these fundamental preparation methods empowers you to use herbs safely and effectively. In the next chapter, we'll explore specific herbs and their benefits in detail. However, if you're eager to start making your own remedies right away, feel free to jump ahead to Part Two.

CHAPTER 5:

ESSENTIAL HERBS AND INGREDIENTS

I go to nature to be soothed and healed, and to have my senses put in order. –John Burroughs

Did you know that natural remedies can help our bodies heal? While herbs form the backbone of most home apothecaries, everyday items like honey, vinegar, salt, and oils can be just as powerful in promoting wellness. In this chapter, we'll take a look at some of the most commonly used herbs and natural ingredients, organizing them by their primary benefits and uses. This section offers a broad overview to help you understand the role of each ingredient in holistic health care. There are more detailed preparation methods and recipes in Part Two, where these ingredients are put into action to address specific ailments.

DIGESTIVE AND GUT HEALTH INGREDIENTS

The digestive system is often the first stop in assessing overall health. Whether it's a case of the post-lunch bloat or the discomfort that accompanies motion sickness, certain herbs and natural ingredients have been lauded for their ability to soothe and support gut health.

PEPPERMINT (*MENTHA X PIPERITA*)

Properties: Cooling, antispasmodic, decongestant

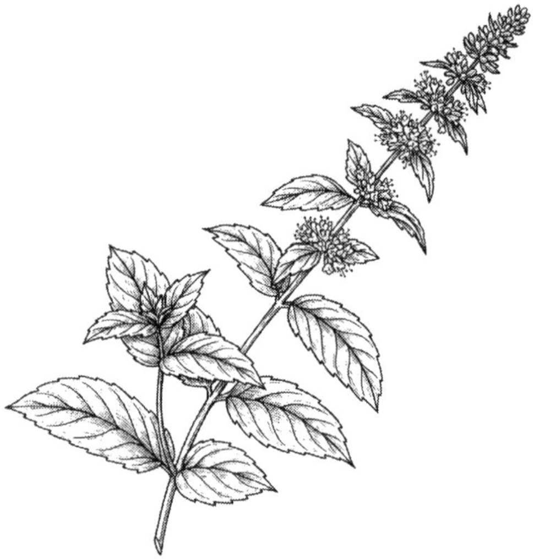

The cooling aroma of peppermint tea wafting through the air is not just refreshing; it actively helps in easing bloating, nausea, and stuffy noses. When consumed, peppermint works by relaxing the muscles of the digestive tract, reducing spasms, and loosening phlegm to provide gentle relief from discomfort.

Warnings and precautions: Do not use peppermint if you're allergic to the mint family or have been diagnosed with gastroesophageal reflux disease (GERD). Also, abstain from using peppermint and peppermint oil on small children, as it may lead to spasms that can interfere with breathing (Peppermint, n.d.).

GINGER (*ZINGIBER OFFICINALE*)

Properties: Warming, anti-inflammatory, antiemetic, carminative, and circulatory stimulant

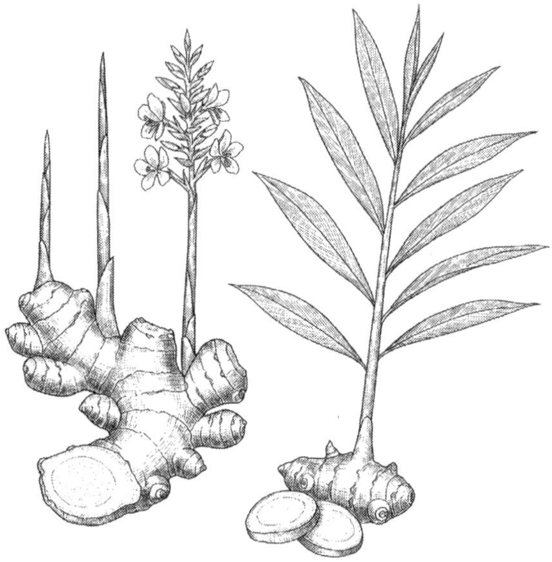

Ginger effectively soothes digestive discomfort, reduces nausea, and supports circulation. Its carminative effects help alleviate bloating and gas, while its antiemetic properties make it a popular remedy for motion sickness and morning

sickness. Additionally, ginger's ability to stimulate circulation can provide relief from cold hands and feet (Kalyan, n.d.).

Warnings and precautions: Ginger is safe for most people in small amounts, but in high doses it can increase the risk of bleeding and affect insulin levels. People with gallbladder issues are advised to use ginger very cautiously. Also, if you're on certain medications (beta-blockers, anticoagulants, and diabetes medications), it's best to consult a healthcare provider before using ginger as it may interact with these medications (Modi & Modi, 2021).

FENNEL (*FOENICULUM VULGARE*)

Properties: Carminative, antispasmodic, anti-inflammatory, diuretic, and antioxidant

Fennel seeds are well-known for their carminative properties, which means they help in preventing gas formation. By relaxing the gastrointestinal muscles, fennel can effectively prevent stomach cramps and minimize flatulence. This makes fennel tea a great ally for those struggling with digestive discomforts (and those who live with them!).

Warnings and precautions: Do not use if you are allergic to the carrot family. Fennel may interact with tamoxifen (a cancer drug) (Braveman, 2024). Be careful of large doses of fennel as it may not be safe for pregnant or breastfeeding women.

GERMAN CHAMOMILE (*MATRICARIA CHAMOMILLA*)

Properties: Anti-inflammatory, anti-spasmodic, calming, and analgesic

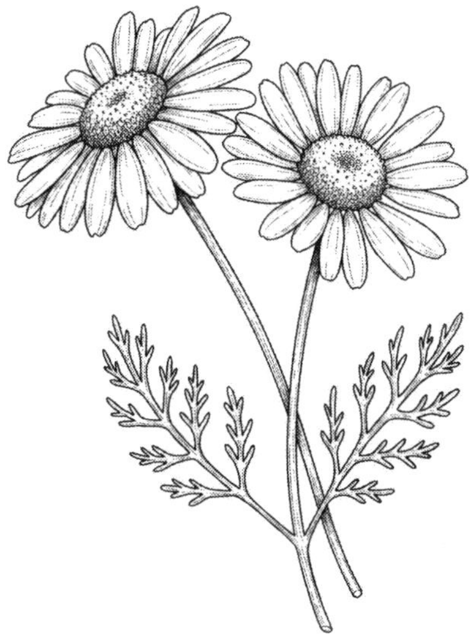

Chamomile tea's popularity is often attributed to its anti-inflammatory effects, particularly beneficial for calming an irritated stomach lining. It's more than just a nightcap drink; it's a gentle healer for the digestive tract. Chamomile can help bring relief to indigestion and gas, while giving your gut a helping hand overall.

Warnings and precautions: Be cautious of using this herb if you are allergic to the ragweed family. Do not use chamomile if you are going to drive or perform a task that requires a highly focused mind. May interact with sedatives, hormonal treatments, and blood-thinning medications, so seek medical advice before using (*German Chamomile*, n.d.).

SLIPPERY ELM (*ULMUS RUBRA*)

Properties: Soothing, protective, and anti-inflammatory

Slippery elm is known for its mucilage content, which forms a soothing gel when mixed with water, helping to coat and protect the digestive tract. This protective layer can relieve symptoms of acid reflux, gastritis, and other digestive discomforts while reducing inflammation in the gut lining.

Warnings and precautions: Slippery elm is generally safe for most people, but it may interfere with the absorption of medications if taken simultaneously.

LICORICE ROOT (*GLYCYRRHIZA GLABRA*)

Properties: Soothing, anti-inflammatory, and demulcent

Licorice root is well-regarded for its ability to soothe the digestive tract by forming a protective coating over irritated mucous membranes. It is particularly effective in managing symptoms of acid reflux, heartburn, and stomach ulcers, thanks to its anti-inflammatory properties. The demulcent action helps to ease discomfort and promote healing of the stomach lining.

Warnings and precautions: Using licorice root for long periods can have serious side effects, such as elevated blood pressure.

APPLE CIDER VINEGAR (*MALUS DOMESTICA*)

Properties: Digestive aid, probiotic-supporting, and alkalizing

Apple cider vinegar is often used to support digestion by stimulating stomach acid production and promoting healthy gut bacteria. Its mildly alkalizing effect on the body can help balance pH levels, making it useful for managing symptoms of acid reflux and indigestion.

Warnings and precautions: Consuming apple cider vinegar undiluted can erode tooth enamel and irritate the throat and digestive tract.

IMMUNE-BOOSTING AND RESPIRATORY SUPPORT INGREDIENTS

ECHINACEA (*ECHINACEA PURPUREA*)

Properties: immune-boosting, anti-inflammatory, and antiviral

It is commonly used to help prevent or shorten the duration of colds, support the immune system, reduce inflammation, and promote overall wellness. It also has mild pain-relieving and antioxidant effects.

Warnings and precautions: If you're allergic to members of the ragweed family, it may be prudent to avoid using this plant. People living with autoimmune conditions are not encouraged to use echinacea, as it may worsen symptoms (Echinacea, 2020).

ELDERBERRY (*SAMBUCUS NIGRA*)

Properties: Antiviral, immune-boosting, and flu-fighting

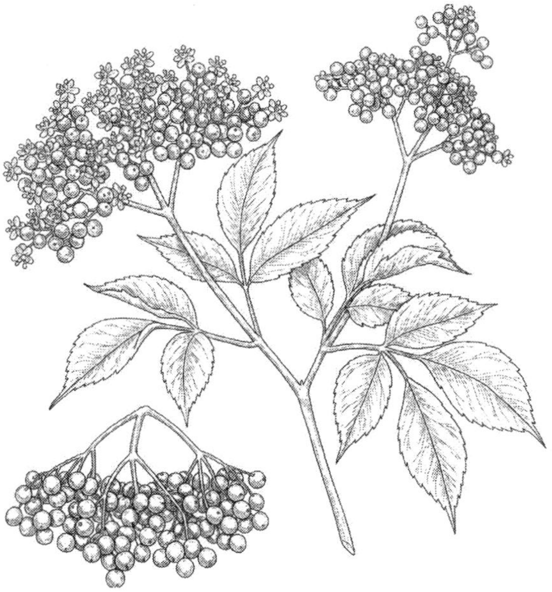

Elderberry is commonly used to support the immune system and combat symptoms of colds and flu. Its antiviral properties help reduce the severity and duration of flu symptoms, and it also promotes overall wellness by boosting immune function.

Warnings and precautions: Elderberry should be consumed only after being properly cooked or prepared, as raw berries and other parts of the plant can be toxic (Elderberry, 2025). People with autoimmune conditions should consult a healthcare provider before using it.

GARLIC (*ALLIUM SATIVUM*)

Properties: Natural antibiotic, immune-boosting, and anti-inflammatory

Garlic has been traditionally used for its powerful natural antibiotic and antimicrobial properties, helping to fight infections and strengthen the immune system. Additionally, garlic's anti-inflammatory effects can support cardiovascular health and overall wellness (Ansary et al., 2020).

Warnings and precautions: Garlic may cause digestive upset or irritation in some people, especially when consumed in large amounts.

THYME (*THYMUS VULGARIS*)

Properties: Mucus-clearing, antimicrobial, and lung-supporting

Thyme is well-known for its ability to clear mucus from the respiratory system, making it effective for easing coughs, colds, and respiratory infections. Its antimicrobial properties help combat infections, and it also supports lung health by relieving inflammation in the airways (Hammoudi Halat et al., 2022).

Warnings and precautions: Thyme is generally safe, but excessive use can cause digestive upset, including nausea or heartburn.

MULLEIN (*VERBASCUM THAPSUS*)

Properties: Soothing, anti-inflammatory, and respiratory-supporting

Mullein is known for its soothing effect on the respiratory tract, helping to relieve coughs, bronchitis, and other respiratory irritations. It has mild anti-inflammatory properties that can reduce swelling in the airways and improve overall lung function (Turker & Gurel, 2005).

Warnings and precautions: Avoid if allergic to plants in the *Scrophulariaceae* family (figworts) as it may cause sensitivities, and pregnant women should consult with a healthcare provider before using it.

ASTRAGALUS (*ASTRAGALUS MEMBRANACEUS*)

Properties: Immune-boosting, anti-inflammatory, and adaptogenic

Astragalus is used to strengthen the immune system, especially for long-term health maintenance. It also helps the body cope with stress and fatigue, and its anti-inflammatory effects support overall vitality and wellness (Meixner, 2024).

Warnings and precautions: Individuals with autoimmune conditions should avoid using astragalus. Those on immunosuppressive drugs should also avoid this herb, as it may interact with these medications.

RAW HONEY (*APIS MELLIFERA*)

Properties: Antiviral, antibacterial, and soothing

Raw honey has natural antiviral and antibacterial properties that make it effective for soothing sore throats, treating coughs, and healing minor wounds. It also supports digestive health.

Warnings and precautions: Raw honey should never be given to infants under one year of age due to the risk of botulism. People with allergies to honey or bee products should avoid it, and excessive consumption of honey may lead to weight gain due to its high sugar content.

PAIN RELIEF AND ANTI-INFLAMMATORY INGREDIENTS

TURMERIC (*CURCUMA LONGA*)

Properties: Anti-inflammatory, antioxidant, and supports joint health

Turmeric is known as a potent anti-inflammatory with antioxidant effects. It not only helps reduce joint pain and stiffness but also supports heart and brain health by combating oxidative stress (Benzie & Wachtel-Galor, 2011).

Warnings and precautions: High doses may cause digestive discomfort, nausea, or dizziness. If you have gallbladder issues or take blood-thinning medications, consult your doctor before use.

WILLOW BARK (*SALIX ALBA*)

Properties: Natural pain reliever, anti-inflammatory

Willow bark contains salicin, a compound similar to aspirin, which helps relieve pain, inflammation, and fevers naturally. It is effective for treating headaches, lower back pain, and arthritis symptoms and is often considered a gentler alternative to synthetic pain relievers. Its anti-inflammatory effects can also support joint health (Whitlock, 2020).

Warnings and precautions: Not recommended for children, pregnant women, or people with aspirin allergies or peptic ulcers.

FEVERFEW (*TANACETUM PARTHENIUM*)

Properties: Anti-inflammatory, migraine prevention

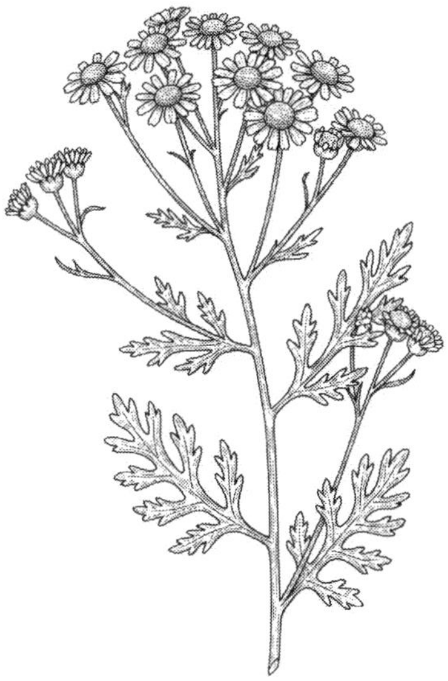

Feverfew is commonly used to prevent migraines and alleviate inflammation. It is used to relieve migraines, arthritis, and menstrual pain (Whitlock, 2020).

Warnings and precautions: Not recommended during pregnancy, as it may cause uterine contractions. Chewing fresh leaves may cause mouth ulcers, and it can interact with blood-thinning and migraine medications.

CAYENNE PEPPER (*CAPSICUM ANNUUM*)

Properties: Stimulates circulation, pain relief

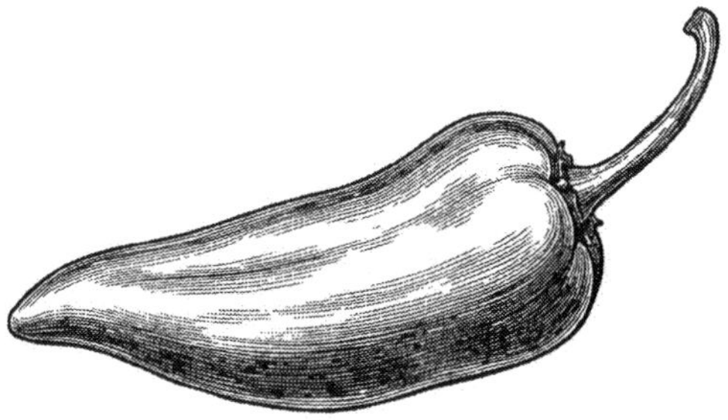

Cayenne pepper contains capsaicin, which promotes circulation and acts as a natural pain reliever by desensitizing nerve receptors. It is particularly effective when applied topically for arthritis, muscle pain, and nerve discomfort.

Warnings and precautions: Use gloves during application and avoid contact with sensitive areas such as the eyes, mucous membranes, or open wounds. Consuming large amounts may cause stomach discomfort.

DEVIL'S CLAW (*HARPAGOPHYTUM PROCUMBENS*)

Properties: Anti-inflammatory, analgesic, supports joint and muscle health

Devil's Claw is known for its ability to reduce inflammation and alleviate muscle and joint pain, particularly in arthritis. This herb is also sometimes used to manage lower back pain.

Warnings and precautions: Not advised for people with stomach ulcers, gallstones, or diabetes. May interact with blood-thinning medications and cause mild digestive upset.

FRANKINCENSE (*BOSWELLIA SERRATA*)

Properties: Anti-inflammatory, supports joint and respiratory health

Boswellia, also called frankincense, is prized for its ability to reduce inflammation, particularly in cases of arthritis and inflammatory bowel conditions. It may also support respiratory health by reducing bronchial inflammation.

Warnings and precautions: May cause digestive upset, such as acid reflux or nausea, in some individuals. Consult a healthcare provider if pregnant or taking medications for inflammation.

EPSOM SALT (*MAGNESIUM SULFATE*)

Properties: Relieves muscle soreness, reduces inflammation, detoxifies

Epsom salt baths can be used to ease muscle soreness, reduce inflammation, and encourage relaxation. The magnesium absorbed through the skin helps soothe cramps and alleviate stress. Regular use may also assist in flushing toxins from the body.

Warnings and precautions: Avoid ingesting Epsom salts unless directed by a healthcare provider, as it can cause digestive distress.

SLEEP AND STRESS-RELIEF INGREDIENTS

LAVENDER (*LAVANDULA ANGUSTIFOLIA*)

Properties: Calming, promotes sleep, anti-anxiety

Lavender is known for having a soothing aroma, which can help with calming the mind, reducing stress, and promoting restful sleep. Its relaxing effects can be used to ease tension headaches and mild anxiety, making it a popular choice for aromatherapy. The best part? Lavender is a very skin-loving herb, making it useful for soothing skin irritations when applied topically (Bowman, 2023).

Warnings and precautions: May cause drowsiness or allergic reactions in some individuals. Avoid excessive use during pregnancy and consult a healthcare provider if taking sedatives or medications for blood pressure.

VALERIAN ROOT (*VALERIANA OFFICINALIS*)

Properties: Natural sedative, aids in insomnia and anxiety relief

Valerian root is often used to support sleep and manage insomnia due to its sedative effects on the nervous system. Its calming properties also make it useful for easing nervous tension and muscle cramps (Valerian, 2020).

Warnings and precautions: May cause drowsiness, dizziness, or digestive upset in some individuals. Avoid using it with alcohol, sedatives, or before operating heavy machinery. Not recommended for long-term use without consulting a healthcare provider. Avoid if you have an allergy to any members of the honeysuckle family.

ASHWAGANDHA (*WITHANIA SOMNIFERA*)

Properties: Adaptogen, helps with stress and adrenal fatigue, supports immune health

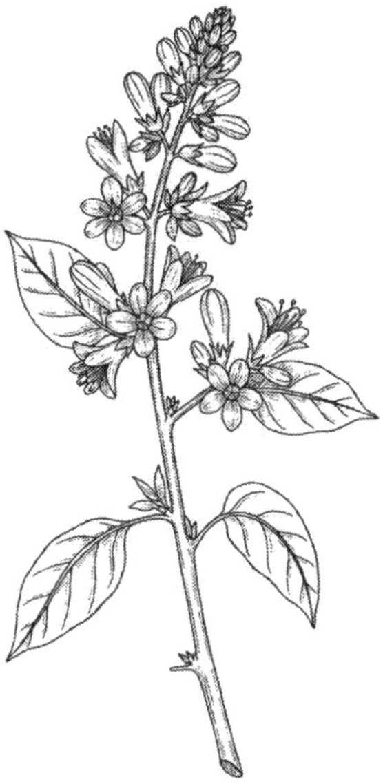

Ashwagandha is an adaptogenic herb that helps the body manage stress by regulating cortisol levels and supporting adrenal function (*Ashwagandha*, 2023). It also enhances energy, focus, and resilience against fatigue.

Warnings and precautions: Not recommended for pregnant women or people with hyperthyroidism. May interact with thyroid, blood sugar, and immunosuppressant medications. Avoid using if you have an allergy to any members of the nightshade family. It's best to speak to your doctor or healthcare provider before use.

LEMON BALM (*MELISSA OFFICINALIS*)

Properties: Reduces anxiety and stress, supports digestion

Lemon balm is a gentle yet effective herb for managing anxiety, stress, and mild insomnia. Its calming effects are believed to help soothe nervousness and may promote mental clarity. The herb is also used to soothe bloating, gas, and cramps.

Warnings and precautions: May interact with thyroid medications and sedatives. Avoid excessive use during pregnancy. Do not use if you are allergic to the mint family. Long-term use without breaks is not recommended.

PASSIONFLOWER (*PASSIFLORA INCARNATA*)

Properties: Aids in deep sleep, reduces anxiety, mild sedative

Passionflower is prized for its ability to promote deep, restful sleep and reduce symptoms of anxiety and nervousness. Its mild sedative effects also make it useful for easing symptoms of insomnia (Ashpari, 2024).

Warnings and precautions: May cause drowsiness or dizziness. Avoid using with sedatives, antidepressants, or during pregnancy without consulting a healthcare provider.

OAT STRAW (*AVENA SATIVA*)

Properties: Supports the nervous system, soothes anxiety, boosts energy

Oat straw is known for its gentle, nourishing effects on the nervous system, making it effective for reducing anxiety and supporting cognitive function (Kennedy et al., 2020).

Warnings and precautions: Generally considered safe, but people with gluten sensitivity should choose certified gluten-free sources. Excessive use may cause mild digestive upset.

MAGNESIUM (*FROM FOOD SOURCES OR EPSOM SALT BATHS*)

Properties: Muscle relaxation, supports sleep quality, reduces stress

Magnesium is essential for muscle and nerve function, and its relaxing effects can help alleviate insomnia, muscle cramps, and stress. Absorbing magnesium through Epsom salt baths or consuming magnesium-rich foods like nuts, seeds, and leafy greens can enhance sleep quality and support heart health. Regular magnesium intake also helps regulate mood and may prevent migraines.

Warnings and precautions: Excessive intake can cause diarrhea, stomach cramps, or irregular heartbeat. If you live with kidney disease, it is best to speak to your doctor before using magnesium or Epsom salts.

SKIN HEALING AND TOPICAL INGREDIENTS

CALENDULA (*CALENDULA OFFICINALIS*)

Properties: Soothes skin, speeds up wound healing, anti-inflammatory

Calendula is a very soothing herb; it is able to calm irritated skin, reduce inflammation, and promote the healing of cuts, scrapes, and minor burns. Its natural antibacterial and antifungal properties also make it effective for treating rashes, eczema, and insect bites.

Warnings and precautions: Generally safe for topical use, but people allergic to plants in the Asteraceae (daisy) family should use caution. Avoid applying to deep wounds without consulting a healthcare provider.

PLANTAIN (*PLANTAGO MAJOR*)

Properties: Reduces itching, promotes skin repair, anti-inflammatory

Plantain leaves have been traditionally used to soothe insect bites, rashes, and minor wounds due to their anti-inflammatory and antimicrobial properties. This remedy can be used as a poultice. The leaves can be infused into oils, which can be used to make salves.

Warnings and precautions: Generally safe, but perform a patch test to ensure no allergic reactions occur. Avoid using it if you have a known allergy to plantain or bananas.

ALOE VERA (*ALOE BARBADENSIS MILLER*)

Properties: Hydrates, soothes burns, anti-inflammatory

Aloe vera cools and hydrates the skin, making it ideal for treating sunburns, minor burns, and dry or irritated skin. Its gel contains vitamins, enzymes, and antioxidants that help reduce inflammation and promote skin healing. Regular use can also help prevent scarring and improve skin elasticity.

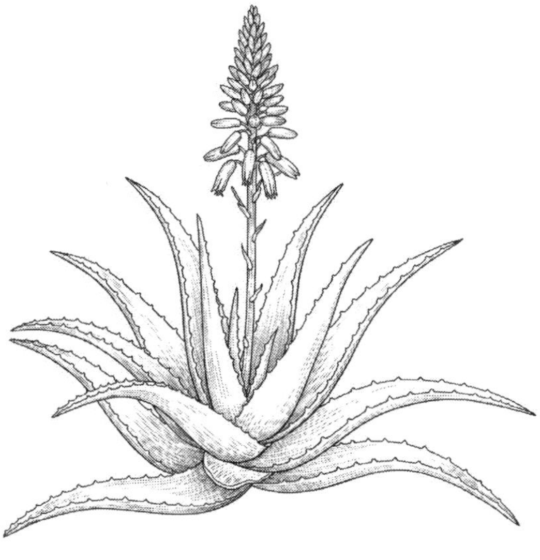

Warnings and precautions: Some individuals may experience allergic reactions; perform a patch test before regular use. Avoid applying to deep wounds.

TEA TREE OIL (*MELALEUCA ALTERNIFOLIA*)

Properties: Antimicrobial, fights acne and infections, anti-inflammatory

Tea tree oil has powerful antibacterial, antiviral, and antifungal properties, making it effective against acne, athlete's foot, and minor skin infections (Carson et al., 2006). Its anti-inflammatory effects also help reduce redness and swelling in blemishes and insect bites.

Warnings and precautions: Should always be diluted before applying to the skin. Avoid use if you are allergic to members of the myrtle family. Not safe for internal use or for pets.

COMFREY (*SYMPHYTUM OFFICINALE*)

Properties: Speeds healing of bruises, sprains, and minor injuries, anti-inflammatory

Traditionally used to promote the healing of bruises and sprains. Can be used in topical applications such as salves, compresses and poultices. Comfrey is believed to help reduce pain and swelling in joints and muscles.

Warnings and precautions: Under no circumstances should comfrey be ingested. Do not apply to deep wounds or broken skin for extended periods.

BAKING SODA (*SODIUM BICARBONATE*)

Properties: Soothes insect bites, rashes, and mild burns, alkaline

Baking soda helps neutralize acidic irritants from insect bites and soothes skin inflammation and itching. When made into a paste with water, it can calm mild burns and reduce discomfort from rashes. It's a gentle exfoliant and can be used to remove dead skin cells.

Warnings and precautions: Avoid using on open wounds or sensitive areas. It can dry the skin out if overused.

COCONUT OIL (*COCOS NUCIFERA*)

Properties: Moisturizes skin, antimicrobial, anti-inflammatory

Coconut oil is highly effective for moisturizing dry skin, reducing inflammation, and supporting wound healing. Its antimicrobial properties can help prevent infections in minor cuts and scrapes.(Wallace, 2019). It also soothes eczema and dermatitis symptoms by creating a protective barrier on the skin.

Warnings and precautions: May clog pores for some skin types. Perform a patch test before using extensively on the face or sensitive areas.

SEA SALT

Properties: Promotes wound healing, natural antiseptic, anti-inflammatory

Sea salt contains minerals that help cleanse wounds, reduce inflammation, and speed up the healing process. Its natural antiseptic properties make it effective for disinfecting minor cuts and preventing infection. Sea salt baths can also soothe irritated skin and support detoxification.

Warnings and precautions: Avoid using on deep wounds or broken skin, as it may cause stinging and irritation. Rinse thoroughly after use to prevent salt buildup on the skin.

WOMEN'S HEALTH AND HORMONE BALANCING INGREDIENTS

RASPBERRY LEAF (*RUBUS IDAEUS*)

Properties: Tones the uterus, supports pregnancy, rich in vitamins and minerals

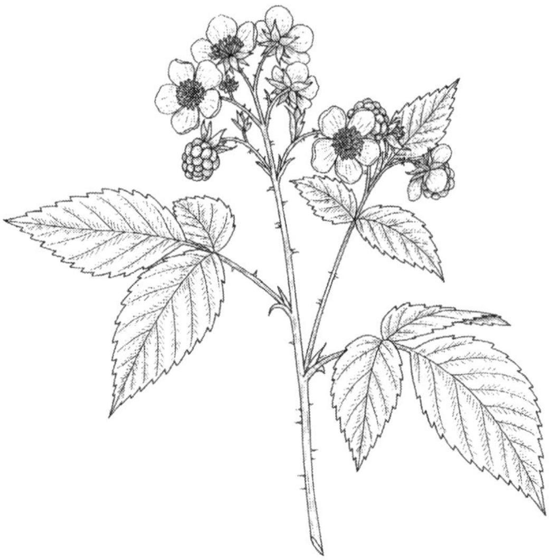

Raspberry leaf is known for its ability to tone the muscles of the uterus, which can be beneficial for

women during pregnancy, particularly in the third trimester, as it may help prepare the body for labor. It's also known to support overall reproductive health, and its high vitamin and mineral content can help nurture the body during pregnancy (Bowman et al., 2021).

Warnings and precautions: Generally safe for use, but it's best to consult a healthcare provider before use. Avoid use if you are allergic to the rose family.

CHASTE TREE (*VITEX AGNUS-CASTUS*)

Properties: Balances hormones, reduces PMS, supports reproductive health

This remedy is widely used to balance hormones and to bring relief to problematic PMS symptoms, such as irritability, mood swings, and bloating. Chaste tree is believed to encourage a healthy menstrual cycle, support fertility, and may help to ease the symptoms of menopause..

Warnings and precautions: Should not be used by women who are pregnant, breastfeeding, or those living with hormone-sensitive conditions. Avoid use if you are allergic to the mint family.

DONG QUAI (*ANGELICA SINENSIS*)

Properties: Eases menstrual cramps, alleviates menopause symptoms, supports blood circulation

Often referred to as "female ginseng," it is traditionally used in Chinese medicine to support women's health. It helps ease menstrual cramps, promotes blood circulation, and can be useful for alleviating symptoms of menopause.

Warnings and precautions: May increase the risk of bleeding, especially when taken with blood-thinning medications.

BLACK COHOSH (*CIMICIFUGA RACEMOSA*)

Properties: Supports hormonal balance in menopause, relieves hot flashes

This remedy is often used to manage and bring relief to symptoms of menopause, particularly hot flashes, mood swings, and night sweats. It helps support hormonal balance, acting on estrogen receptors in the body to reduce menopause-related discomfort.

Warnings and precautions: Should not be used for extended periods without medical supervision. If you're allergic to the buttercup family, avoid usage.

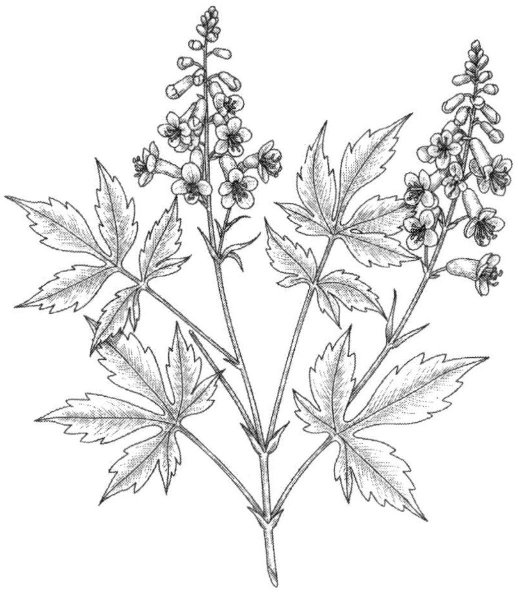

EVENING PRIMROSE OIL (*OENOTHERA BIENNIS*)

Properties: Supports PMS, promotes skin health, rich in omega-6 fatty acids

Evening primrose oil is beneficial for women experiencing PMS or menstrual discomfort, as it helps reduce inflammation and hormonal fluctuations. It is also often used for alleviating symptoms of eczema, acne, and dryness.

Warnings and precautions: People on blood-thinning medications should talk to their healthcare provider before use, as a risk of interaction exists. Also, pregnant women are strongly advised to seek advice from a healthcare professional before use.

FLAXSEEDS (*LINUM USITATISSIMUM*)

Properties: Naturally supports estrogen balance, rich in fiber, and omega-3s

Flaxseeds can help balance estrogen levels in the body. This is believed to be helpful in managing symptoms of PMS and menopause. Additionally, flaxseeds are rich in fiber and omega-3 fatty acids, contributing to overall digestive and heart health.

Warnings and precautions: Flaxseeds should be ground before consumption to ensure proper digestion. Excessive consumption can cause digestive upset, so it's best to start with small amounts.

DETOX AND LIVER-SUPPORTING INGREDIENTS

DANDELION ROOT (*TARAXACUM OFFICINALE*)

Properties: Supports liver function, promotes digestion, acts as a diuretic

Dandelion root is widely known for its ability to aid in digestion. It acts as a natural diuretic, helping the body eliminate excess fluids and toxins, and is often used in detoxification and cleansing routines.

Warnings and precautions: Can interact with diuretic medications and may cause allergic reactions in individuals sensitive to plants in the Asteraceae (daisy) family.

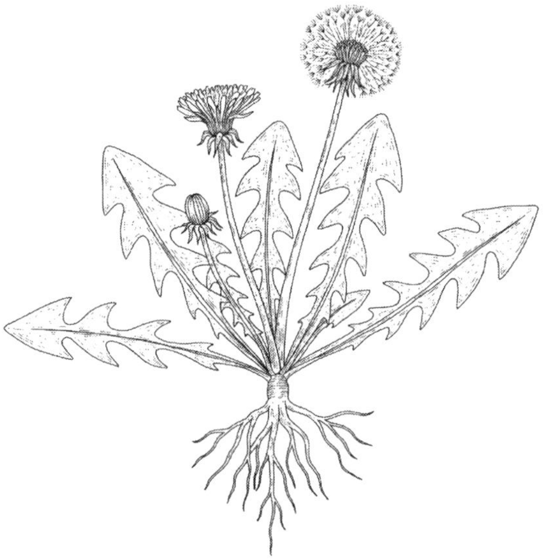

MILK THISTLE (*SILYBUM MARIANUM*)

Properties: Protects the liver from toxins, supports detoxification

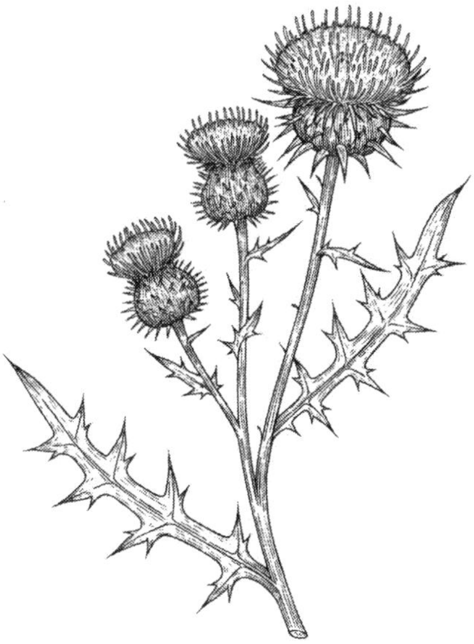

Milk thistle is commonly used to support overall liver function and often features in detox and liver-cleansing regimens.

Warnings and precautions: Generally safe for most people, but those with ragweed allergies or liver disease should use it with caution and consult a healthcare professional before use.

BURDOCK ROOT (*ARCTIUM LAPPA*)

Properties: Helps clear toxins from the bloodstream, promotes skin health

Burdock root is a natural blood purifier, often used to help detoxify the body and promote healthy skin. It supports the elimination of waste and toxins through the kidneys and skin, making it beneficial for conditions like acne and eczema.

Warnings and precautions: It may interact with diabetes medications due to its potential to lower blood sugar levels.

NETTLE (*URTICA DIOICA*)

Properties: Supports kidney function, provides essential minerals, acts as a detoxifier

Nettle is rich in vitamins and minerals, including iron, calcium, and magnesium, which contribute to overall wellness. Nettle is believed (and is often used) to help the body detox in a natural and gentle way.

Warnings and precautions: May interact with blood-thinning medications and diuretics.

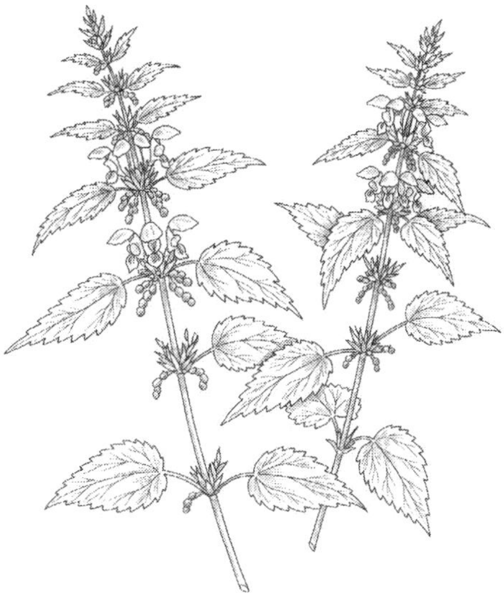

LEMON (*CITRUS LIMON*)

Properties: Supports detoxification, promotes liver function, high in vitamin C

The high vitamin C content helps boost the immune system and promotes the body's natural detoxification processes.

Warnings and precautions: While lemon is generally safe, it may irritate the mouth and stomach if consumed in excess or on an empty stomach. People with citrus allergies should avoid it.

ACTIVATED CHARCOAL

Properties: Aids in removing toxins from the body, supports digestive health

Activated charcoal is commonly used as an emergency treatment for poisoning, as it binds to toxins in the digestive system and prevents them from being absorbed.

Warnings and precautions: Should be used with caution, as it can interfere with the absorption of medications and nutrients.

EVERYDAY NATURAL INGREDIENTS FOR HEALING

MANUKA HONEY (*LEPTOSPERMUM SCOPARIUM*)

Properties: Antimicrobial, soothes sore throats, promotes wound healing

This honey is believed to have powerful antimicrobial properties and can be used to soothe sore throats, encourage wound healing, and support gut health.

Warnings and precautions: While generally safe, those allergic to bee products should avoid it.

HIMALAYAN PINK SALT (*HIMALAYAN SALT*)

Properties: Rich in minerals, supports hydration, balances electrolytes

Himalayan pink salt is a natural salt rich in essential minerals. It can support hydration, balance electrolytes, and even soothe muscle cramps when added to a bath or consumed in moderation.

Warnings and precautions: Individuals with kidney problems or those on a low-sodium diet should use it cautiously.

MAGNESIUM CHLORIDE (*MAGNESIUM CHLORIDE FLAKES*)

Properties: Supports muscle relaxation, detoxification, and aids in skin hydration

Magnesium chloride is a form of magnesium that can be absorbed through the skin, making it popular for soaking in baths to relieve muscle cramps and promote relaxation. It also supports skin hydration and detoxification.

Warnings and precautions: Should not be consumed. Those with kidney disease should consult a healthcare provider before using magnesium supplements or baths.

WHITE VINEGAR (*ACETIC ACID*)

Properties: Supports digestion, balances stomach acidity, antimicrobial

White vinegar can be used in place of apple cider vinegar, offering similar benefits in supporting digestion and balancing stomach acid levels. It also works as a natural disinfectant. Though it doesn't have the same nutritional profile, it can still be effective for digestive and health-related uses.

Warnings and precautions: Due to its acidity, it may irritate the digestive system or throat if consumed undiluted.

In addition to the healing herbs we previously discussed, other powerful ingredients include honey, apple cider vinegar, baking soda, lemon, coconut oil, and sea salt. Now that you have a well-rounded understanding of these natural remedies, the next step is learning how to harness their benefits. In Part Two, we'll put these ingredients to work by crafting teas, tinctures, salves, and more!

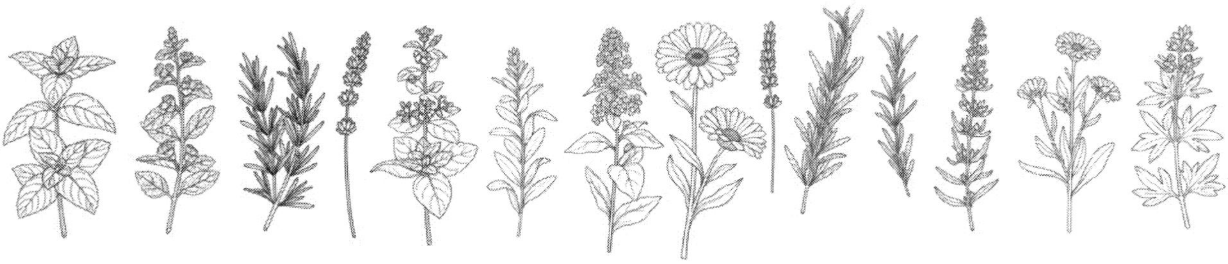

PART TWO:

NATURAL REMEDIES FOR COMMON AILMENTS

CHAPTER 6:

COLD, FLU, AND IMMUNE SUPPORT

When cold and flu season strikes, natural remedies can provide relief and strengthen the immune system. There are trusted herbal and holistic solutions to ease symptoms, shorten recovery time, and fortify your body's natural defenses. From immune-boosting tonics to soothing teas, these remedies harness the power of nature to help you stay resilient against seasonal illnesses.

COLD AND FLU: HERBAL TEAS FOR SYMPTOM RELIEF

Warm herbal teas are a great way to soothe sore throats, ease congestion, and keep your body hydrated – all while giving your immune system a helping hand. The teas in this section are easy to prepare:

GINGER TEA

Relieves congestion, soothes sore throats, and reduces inflammation.

Ingredients:

- 2 cups water
- 1-inch piece fresh ginger, thinly sliced
- 1 tbsp honey (optional)
- ½ lemon, juiced

Instructions:

- Simmer the ginger for 10 minutes to create a strong, fragrant infusion. Then remove from the heat, strain, and stir in honey (if using) and lemon juice. It's best to drink this remedy warm, but don't exceed three cups a day.

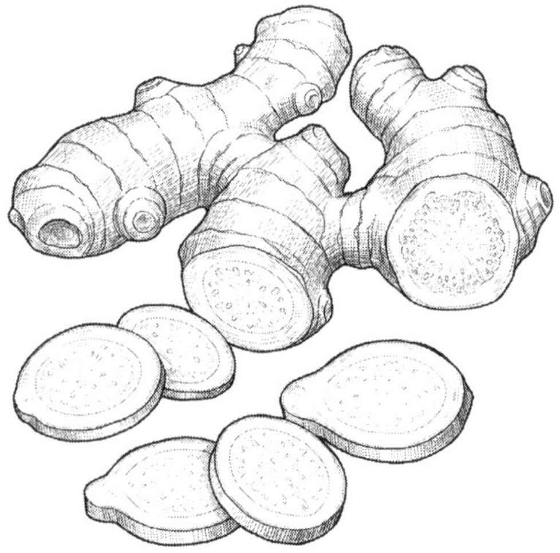

ELDERBERRY TEA

Packed with antiviral properties to help shorten colds and flu.

Ingredients:

- 2 cups water
- 2 tbsp dried elderberries
- 1 tsp cinnamon (optional)
- 1 tbsp honey (optional)

Instructions:

- Simmer elderberries and cinnamon for 15 minutes. Remove from the heat and strain. Stir in the honey and drink warm twice a day.

PEPPERMINT TEAWATER

Clears nasal congestion and reduces fever-related discomfort.

Ingredients:

- 1 cup hot water
- 1 tbsp dried peppermint leaves (or 2 tbsp fresh leaves)
- 1 tsp honey (optional)

Instructions:

- Using hot water, steep the peppermint while covered for 5-7 minutes. Strain and stir the honey in. Drink warm as needed.

ECHINACEA TEA

Boosts immunity and helps fight infections.

Ingredients:

- 1 tsp echinacea root (dried) or echinacea flowers
- 1 cup hot water

Instructions:

- Steep the root or flowers, covered, for 10-15 minutes. Afterward, strain the infusion and drink it warm. You can sweeten with honey if desired. It is advisable not to drink more than three cups of this tea in a day.

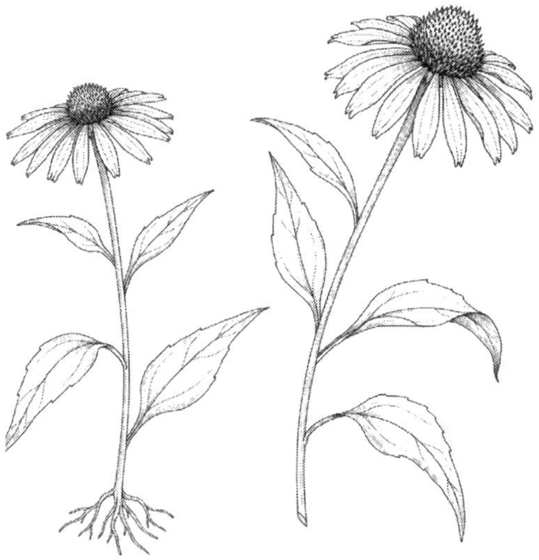

TURMERIC AND BLACK PEPPER TEA

May help support respiratory health and can combat inflammation.

Ingredients:

- 1 teaspoon turmeric powder
- 1 cup hot water
- a pinch of black pepper
- 1 teaspoon lemon juice (optional)

Instructions:

- Using hot water, mix the turmeric powder until completely incorporated. Add the lemon juice and black pepper, then stir to create a homogenous mixture. Drink warm to relieve cold symptoms. Do not drink more than one cup a day.

LEMON BALM AND HONEY TEA

Calms fever, soothes sore throats, and supports relaxation.

Ingredients:

- 1–2 tsp dried (or fresh) lemon balm leaves
- 1 cup hot water
- 1 tsp honey

Instructions:

- Use hot, but not boiling, water to steep the lemon balm for roughly 10 minutes. Strain and stir in honey. Drink warm water at night to ease flu symptoms and promote rest.

COUGH AND SORE THROAT: HONEY-BASED COUGH SYRUPS

Honey has natural antimicrobial properties and coats the throat, making it an ideal base to create cough syrups.

HONEY AND LEMON SYRUP

Calms coughing and relieves throat irritation.

Ingredients

- ½ cup honey
- ¼ cup fresh lemon juice

Instructions

- Mix honey and lemon juice in a jar. Take one teaspoon as needed to relieve coughs. Store the mixture in the fridge for up to a week.

HONEY AND CINNAMON SYRUP

Eases throat irritation and fights infection.

Ingredients

- ½ cup honey
- 1 teaspoon ground cinnamon

Instructions

- Stir cinnamon into the honey until well combined. Take one teaspoon three times a day. The mixture will last up to two weeks when stored at room temperature.

HONEY AND GINGER SYRUP

Reduces throat inflammation and helps loosen mucus.

Ingredients

- ½ cup honey
- 1 tbsp grated fresh ginger

Instructions

- Mix honey and ginger in a jar and let sit for at least two hours. Strain the ginger pieces out and take one teaspoon as needed for sore throat relief. Store the mixture in the refrigerator for up to one week.

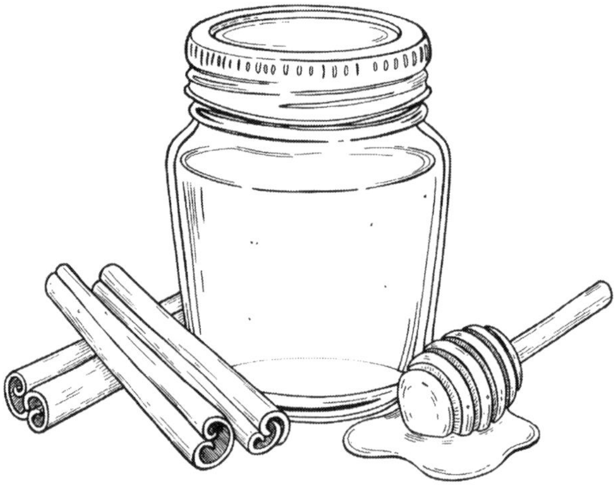

HONEY AND THYME SYRUP

Soothes coughs and supports respiratory health.

Ingredients

- ½ cup honey
- 2 tablespoons dried thyme
- ½ cup hot water

Instructions

- Use hot water to steep the herb (while covered) for 15 minutes. Strain the infusion. Mix the thyme infusion with honey in a jar. Take a teaspoon as needed for cough relief and store the remainder of the syrup in the fridge for up to a week.

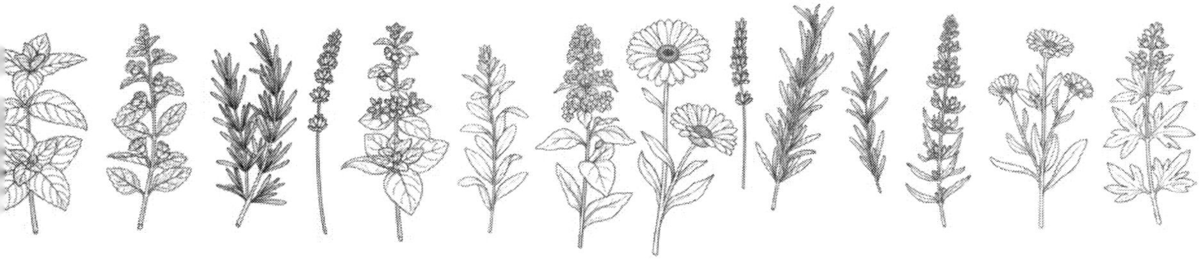

NASAL CONGESTION: STEAM INHALATION REMEDIES

Steam inhalations are a gentle and effective way to open airways, reduce mucus buildup, and alleviate sinus pressure.

EUCALYPTUS STEAM INHALATION

Clears nasal passages and reduces sinus congestion.

Ingredients

- 4 cups boiling water
- 3–5 drops eucalyptus essential oil

Instructions

- Pour piping hot water into a large vessel or bowl. Add eucalyptus oil, stir, and lean over the bowl with a towel over your head. Inhale deeply for 5–10 minutes. Repeat up to twice a day as needed.

PEPPERMINT STEAM INHALATION

Clears nasal congestion and soothes headaches.

Ingredients

- 4 cups hot water
- 5 drops peppermint essential oil or a big handful of fresh peppermint leaves

Instructions

- Pour hot water into a large bowl. Add peppermint essential oil or fresh peppermint leaves. Trap the steam using a towel, and breathe the vapors in for 10 minutes. Repeat as needed for congestion relief.

CHAMOMILE STEAM INHALATION

Gentle and anti-inflammatory for blocked sinuses.

Ingredients

- 4 cups boiling water
- 2 tbsp dried chamomile flowers

Instructions

- Pour piping hot water into a large vessel or bowl. Add the chamomile flowers, then cover your head with a towel to trap the steam. Be careful not to burn as you inhale the steam for up to 10 minutes. Repeat as needed.

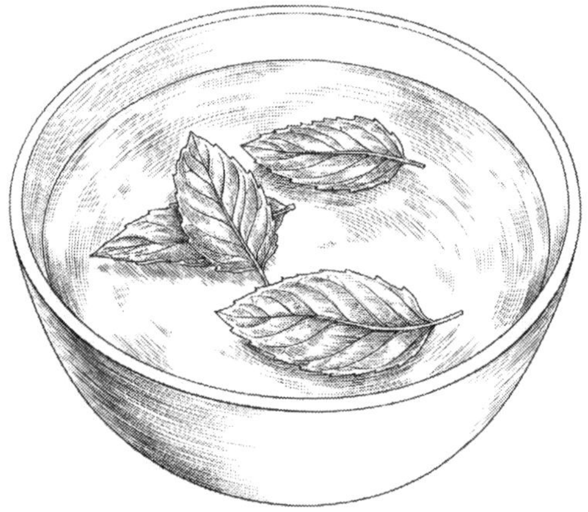

THYME AND ROSEMARY STEAM INHALATION

Supports respiratory health and relieves sinus pressure.

Ingredients

- 4 cups hot water
- 1 tablespoon of thyme (dried or fresh)
- 1 tablespoon of rosemary (dried or fresh)

Instructions

- Add thyme and rosemary to hot water in a bowl. Use a large towel to trap the stream by draping it over your head. Inhale the steam deeply for 10 minutes. Repeat as needed to ease breathing and clear sinuses.

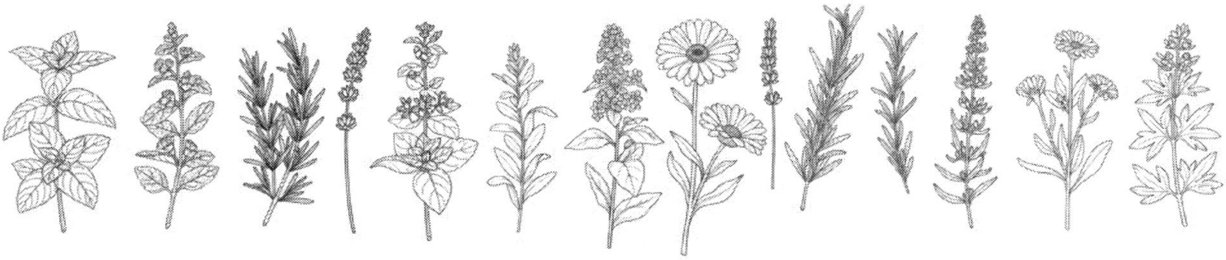

IMMUNE WEAKNESS: HERBAL TINCTURES FOR PREVENTION AND RECOVERY

The tinctures in this section have a long shelf life, making them incredibly handy when cold and flu season arrives. These tinctures can be used to strengthen the immune system and to reduce the duration and intensity of common illnesses like colds and flu.

ECHINACEA TINCTURE

Stimulates the immune system at the onset of cold symptoms.

Ingredients

- 1 cup dried echinacea root
- 2 cups vodka (or apple cider vinegar for an alcohol-free version)

Instructions

- Place echinacea root in a glass jar and cover with vodka or vinegar. Store the jar (sealed) in a dark place for up to six weeks (minimum four) and don't forget to agitate the contents occasionally. Strain the liquid into a dropper bottle. Take one dropperful (about 30 drops) up to three times daily at the first sign of illness.

REISHI MUSHROOM TINCTURE

Enhances immune resilience and reduces inflammation.

Ingredients

- 1 cup dried reishi mushroom slices
- 2 cups vodka (or brandy)
- glass jar with a lid

Instructions

- Follow the same process as with the elderberry tincture. Strain out the mushrooms after six weeks and transfer the liquid to a dropper bottle. Do not exceed a dosage of two dropperfuls per day.

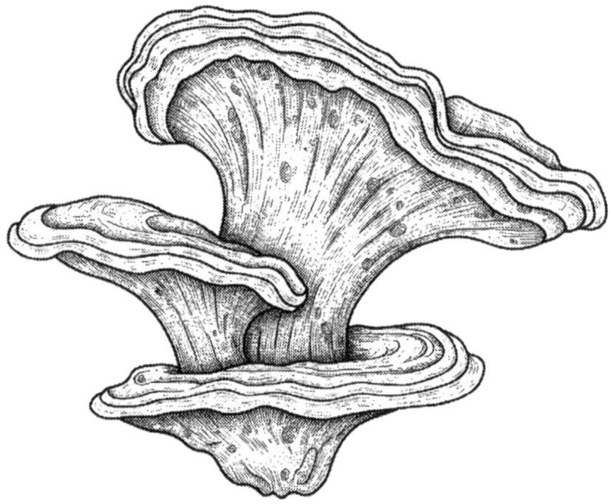

ELDERBERRY TINCTURE

Boosts immune function and helps fight colds and flu.

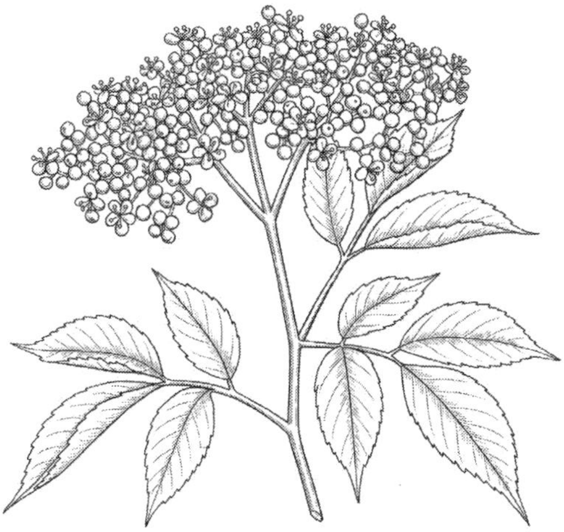

Ingredients

- 1 cup dried elderberries
- 2 cups vodka (or brandy)
- glass jar with a lid

Instructions

- Follow the standard tincture creation process. Ensure the berries are completely covered by the vodka and store in a place away from direct light and heat. Allow a steeping time of four to six weeks, then strain the tincture and transfer it into a dropper bottle. To use, take a teaspoon up to three times a day when you are feeling sick.

ASTRAGALUS TINCTURE

Supports long-term immune health and illness prevention.

Ingredients

- 1 cup dried astragalus root
- 2 cups vodka (or apple cider vinegar)

Instructions

- Follow the same procedure as detailed with the echinacea tincture. When the tincture is ready, take a dropperful daily for immune support.

FEVER AND BODY ACHES: HERBAL BATHS FOR COMFORT

Herbal baths can be used to relieve aches, manage fever, or as part of a detox regimen.

GINGER BATH

Encourages sweating to support detoxification.

Ingredients

- ½ cup freshly grated ginger

Instructions

- Add grated ginger to a warm bath. Soak for 20 minutes and drink plenty of water after the bath.

EUCALYPTUS AND LAVENDER BATH

Relaxes muscles and eases congestion.

Ingredients

- 5 drops of eucalyptus essential oil
- 5 drops of lavender essential oil

Instructions

- Add essential oils to warm bathwater. Soak for 20 minutes and inhale the fragrance deeply.

PEPPERMINT AND ROSEMARY BATH

Relieves body aches and promotes relaxation.

Ingredients

- ½ cup dried peppermint leaves
- ½ cup dried rosemary leaves
- 4 cups boiling water

Instructions

- Create a strong infusion with the peppermint and rosemary. Strain and pour into a warm bath. Soak for at least 20 minutes to ease muscle tension and promote circulation.

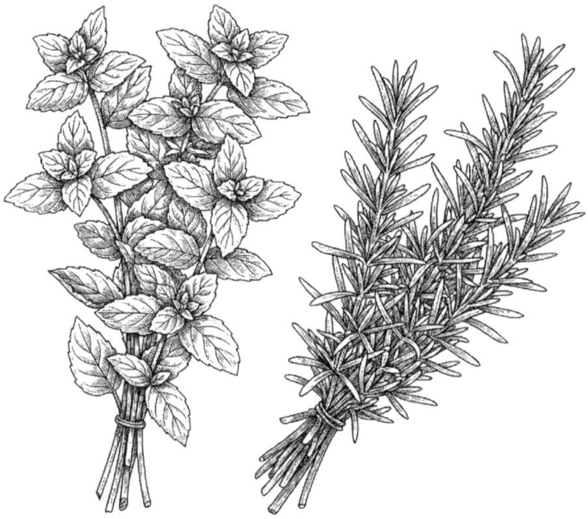

CHAMOMILE AND EPSOM SALT BATH

A calming bath that soothes sore muscles.

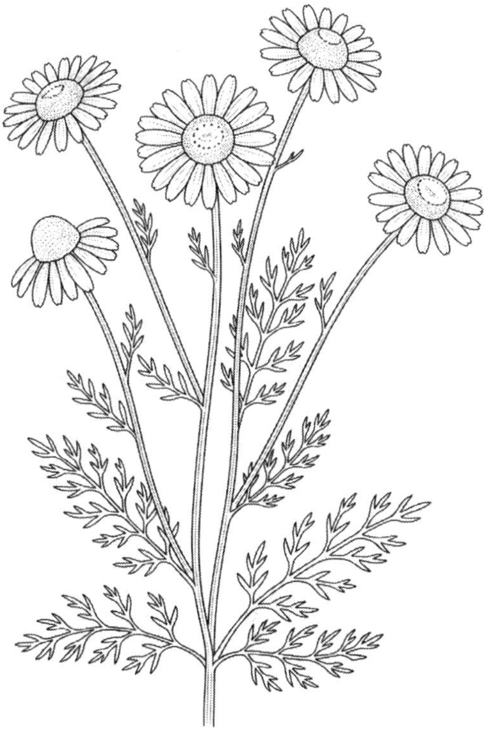

Ingredients

- ½ cup dried chamomile flowers
- 1 cup Epsom salt
- 4 cups boiling water

Instructions

- Make a strong infusion with the chamomile flowers. Pour the strained liquid and Epsom salts into a warm bath. Soak in the bath for 20 minutes.

IMMUNE SUPPORT: HERBAL INFUSED HONEY FOR DAILY USE

Infusing honey with immune-boosting herbs enhances its medicinal properties.

GARLIC INFUSED HONEY

A powerful antimicrobial remedy for daily immune support.

Ingredients

- ½ cup raw honey
- 5 cloves garlic, crushed

Instructions

- Use a clean glass jar and place the crushed garlic in it. Cover the contents with honey. Let it sit for at least three days before using. Take one teaspoon daily or as needed.

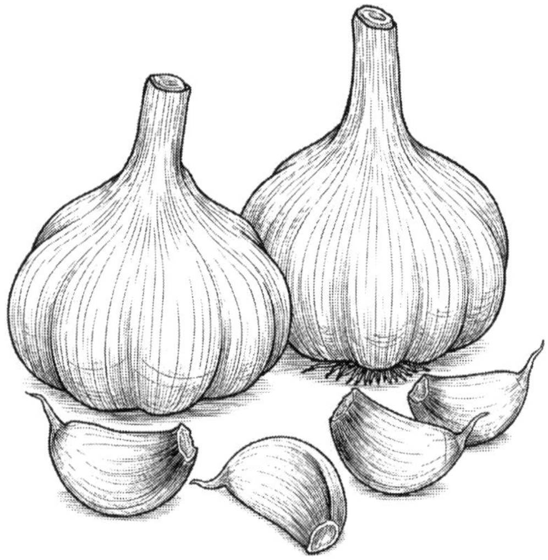

THYME INFUSED HONEY

Supports respiratory health and soothes coughs.

Ingredients

- ½ cup raw honey
- 2 tbsp fresh thyme leaves

Instructions

- Mix thyme and honey in a jar. Let the mixture infuse for five days. Take one teaspoon as needed for cough relief.

LEMON AND ROSEMARY HONEY

Supports respiratory health and boosts immunity.

Ingredients

- ½ cup fresh lemon slices (organic, thinly sliced)
- 2 sprigs fresh rosemary
- 1 cup honey

Instructions

- Place lemon slices and rosemary sprigs in a clean jar. Pour honey over the ingredients, ensuring they are fully submerged. Allow an infusion time of at least one week. Don't forget to stir once a day to help with the extraction process. After the infusion period is done, you can use a teaspoon in warm water or tea daily.

CLOVE AND ORANGE HONEY

Supports immune function and soothes sore throats.

Ingredients

- ½ cup fresh orange zest (organic)
- 5 whole cloves
- a cup of honey

Instructions

Place orange zest and cloves in a clean jar. Pour honey over the ingredients, ensuring they are fully submerged. Allow the mixture to steep for one week. Take a teaspoon daily or mix into warm beverages.

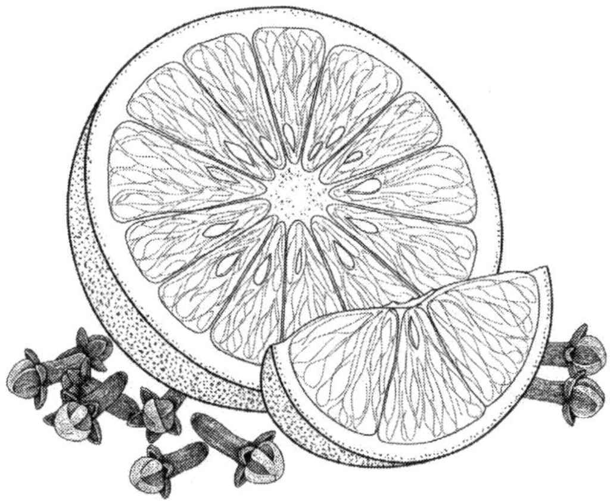

CHAPTER 7:

GUT HEALTH AND DETOX

Your gut does so much for you – it helps you digest food, absorb nutrients, support your immune system, and clear out toxins. There is a growing body of research that's teaching us new things about the importance of gut health, but we already have a wealth of trusted natural remedies passed down to keep your digestion running smoothly and help your body detox gently. These herbal remedies can improve digestion, support your body's natural detox process, and keep your gut microbiome balanced. Whether you're looking for relief from bloating, better nutrient absorption, or a simple reset, these remedies have you covered!

INDIGESTION AND BLOATING: HERBAL TEAS FOR DIGESTIVE COMFORT

Herbal teas can gently relieve indigestion, combat bloating, and soothe the digestive tract.

PEPPERMINT TEA

Relaxes gastrointestinal muscles and relieves gas. See Chapter Six for detailed brewing instructions.

GINGER TEA

Stimulates digestion and reduces bloating.

Ingredients

- 2 cups water
- 1-inch piece fresh ginger, sliced
- 1 tbsp honey (optional)
- ½ lemon, juiced

Instructions

- Bring water to a boil, then add ginger slices. Simmer for 10 minutes, strain, and stir in honey and lemon juice. Drink warm, up to two times daily.

FENNEL SEED TEA

Relaxes intestinal muscles and alleviates gas.

Ingredients

- 1 cup hot water
- 1 tsp crushed fennel seeds

Instructions

- Steep the seeds using hot, not boiling, water for at least 10 minutes. Strain and drink warm after meals.

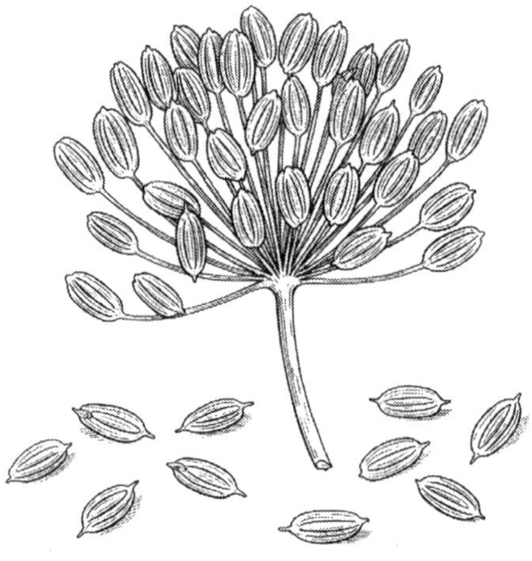

LEMON BALM AND ANISE TEA

Relieves bloating and soothes digestive discomfort.

Ingredients

- 1 teaspoon dried or fresh lemon balm leaves
- ½ teaspoon anise seeds
- 1 cup hot water

Instructions

- Use hot, but not boiling water, to steep the lemon balm and anise seeds. Cover the contents and allow a steeping time of 10 minutes. Strain the infusion and drink it warm after your dinner.

CARAWAY AND LEMON PEEL TEA

Eases bloating and supports digestion.

Ingredients

- 1 teaspoon crushed caraway seeds
- 1 teaspoon dried lemon peel
- 1 cup hot water

Instructions

- Add caraway seeds and lemon peel to a cup. Steep, covered, in hot water for 10 minutes. Then strain the infusion and drink after meals.

CARDAMOM AND CORIANDER TEA

Supports digestion and reduces gas.

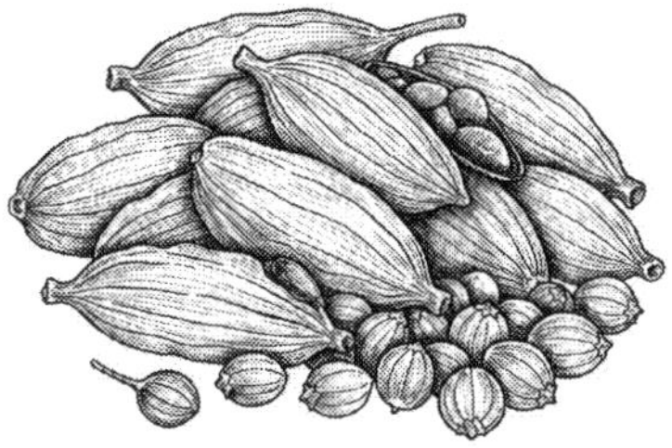

Ingredients

- ½ teaspoon crushed cardamom pods
- ½ teaspoon coriander seeds
- 1 cup hot water

Instructions

- Add the seeds to a teapot. Pour hot, not boiling, water over and cover for 10 minutes while steeping. Strain and drink the infusion warm after meals.

CONSTIPATION: NATURAL LAXATIVE REMEDIES

Over-the-counter constipation medications can sometimes feel harsh on our bodies, but the remedies in this section are designed to gently stimulate bowel movements for predictable relief.

SENNA LEAF TEA

Mild natural laxative for occasional constipation.

Ingredients

- 1 cup hot water
- ½ tsp dried senna leaves

Instructions

- Use hot water and steep the leaves in a covered cup or teapot for five minutes. Strain and drink before bedtime. Use no more than two to three times per week to avoid dependence.

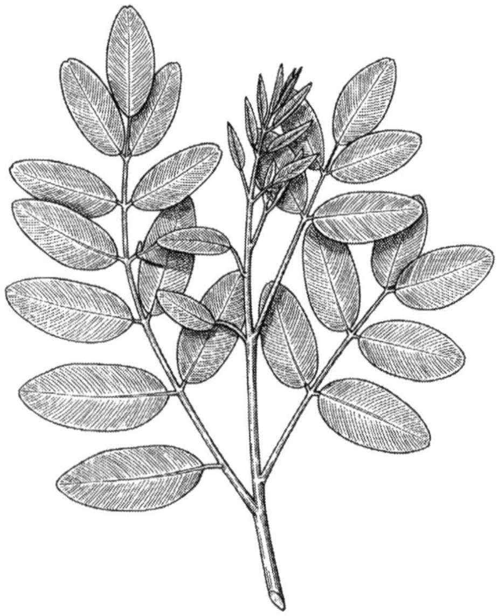

ALOE VERA JUICE

Lubricates the intestines for smoother digestion.

Ingredients

- ¼ cup pure aloe vera juice
- ¾ cup water
- 1 tsp honey (optional)

Instructions

- Mix all the ingredients in a cup until fully incorporated. Drink before breakfast.

WARM LEMON WATER

Stimulates digestion and promotes regular bowel movements.

Ingredients

- 1 cup warm water
- ½ fresh lemon, juiced
- 1 teaspoon honey (optional)

Instructions

- Squeeze fresh lemon juice into a cup of warm water. Stir well and add honey if desired. Drink first thing in the morning on an empty stomach for best results.

PRUNE TEA

Encourages gentle bowel movements and supports digestion.

Ingredients

- 3 dried prunes, chopped
- 1 cup hot water

Instructions

- Add chopped prunes to a cup of hot water. Allow the prunes to infuse for 10-15 minutes, then strain and drink the liquid warm. Drink once daily for relief. In more severe cases, the steeped prunes can be consumed after drinking the tea.

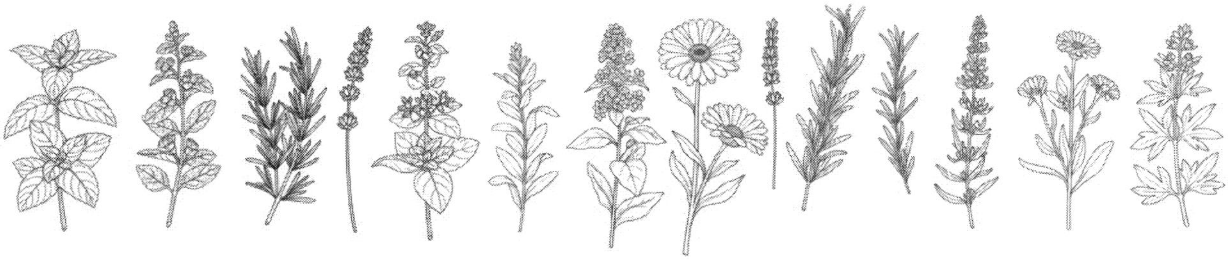

LEAKY GUT SYNDROME: HERBAL REMEDIES FOR GUT LINING REPAIR

These herbs help repair the intestinal lining and reduce inflammation.

SLIPPERY ELM TEA

Coats and soothes the digestive tract, promoting healing.

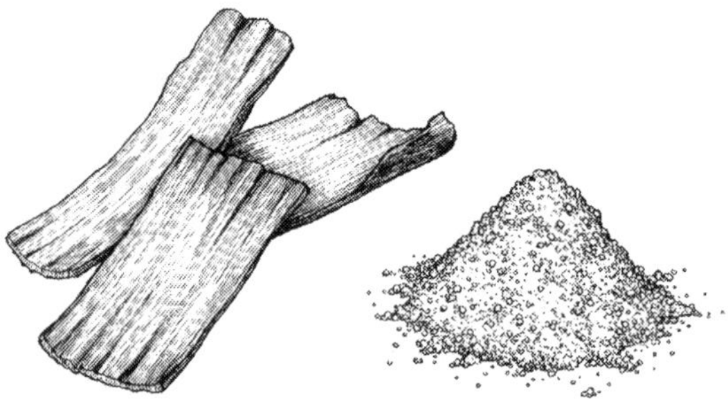

Ingredients

- 1 cup warm water
- 1 tsp slippery elm powder

Instructions

- Combine the herb with warm water to form a homogenous mixture. Drink immediately, up to two times daily.

LICORICE ROOT TEA

Supports mucosal lining repair and reduces inflammation.

Ingredients

- 1 cup hot water
- 1 tsp dried licorice root

Instructions

- Use hot (not boiling) water to steep the herb for 10 minutes. Strain and drink warm.

GREEN TEA

Rich in antioxidants, it helps reduce gut inflammation and supports overall digestive health.

Ingredients

- 1 cup hot water
- 1 green tea bag or 1 tsp loose green tea leaves

Instructions

Steep green tea in hot water for 3–5 minutes. Strain and drink warm. Enjoy up to two cups daily to support gut repair and reduce inflammation.

MARSHMALLOW ROOT TEA

Marshmallow root helps soothe and repair the gut lining by forming a protective layer on the digestive tract.

Ingredients

- 1 cup cold water
- 1 tsp dried marshmallow root

Instructions

- Place marshmallow root in cold water and let it steep for 4–8 hours (or overnight for a stronger infusion). Strain and drink. Drink up to two cups daily to support gut lining repair and reduce inflammation.

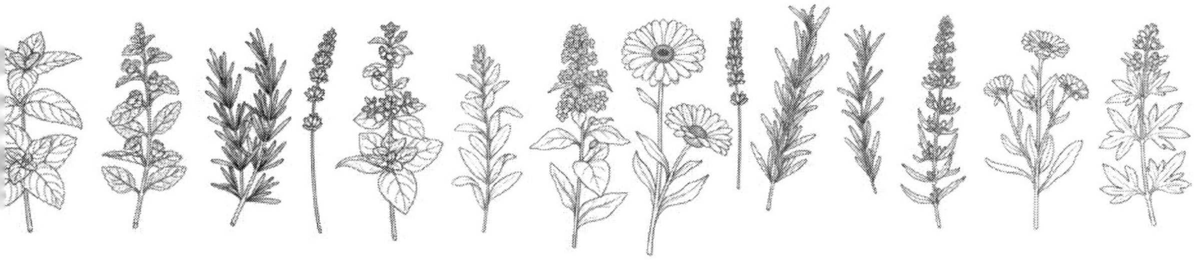

GENERAL DETOXIFICATION: HERBAL TEAS TO SUPPORT DETOX

These herbal teas give your liver and kidneys a natural boost, helping them flush out toxins and keep your body feeling its best.

DANDELION ROOT TEA

Supports liver detoxification and acts as a diuretic.

Ingredients

- 2 cups water
- 1 tbsp dried dandelion root

Instructions

- Simmer the herb for 10 minutes in a small pot, ensuring the lid is on the pot to trap beneficial compounds. Strain the liquid and drink warm.

NETTLE LEAF TEA

Supports detoxification by promoting kidney function and flushing out toxins.

Ingredients

- 1 cup hot water
- 1 tsp dried nettle leaves

Instructions

- Using hot water, steep the herb for 10 minutes while covered. Strain and drink warm. Enjoy one cup daily for gentle detox support.

BURDOCK ROOT TEA

Purifies the blood and supports kidney function.

Ingredients

- 2 cups water
- 1 tbsp dried burdock root

Instructions

- Follow the same procedure as with dandelion root tea. Drink warm.

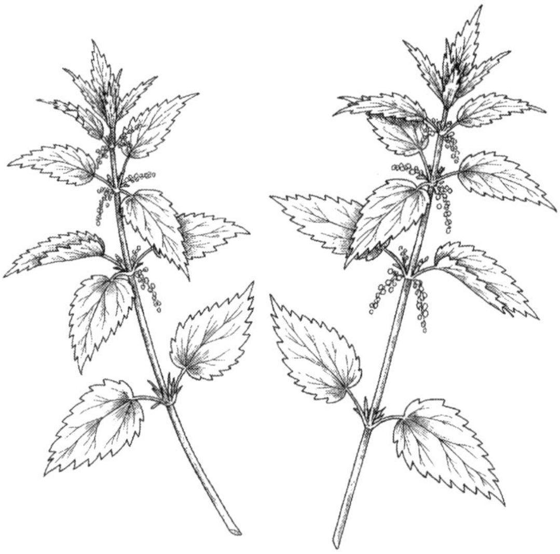

MILK THISTLE TEA

Helps cleanse the liver and supports overall detoxification.

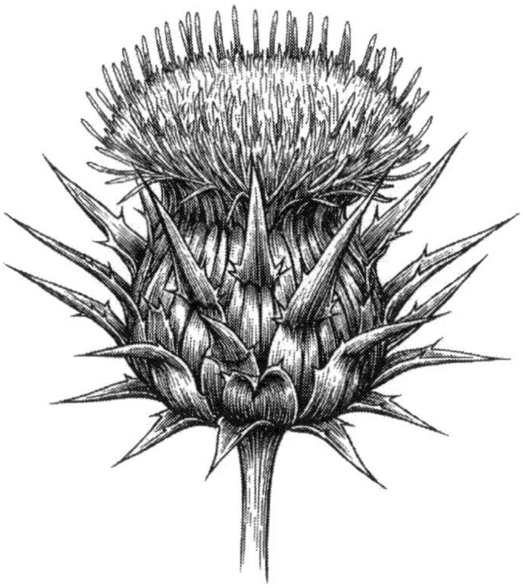

Ingredients

- 1 cup hot water
- 1 tsp crushed milk thistle seeds

Instructions

- Steep the seeds in hot (not boiling) water for 15 minutes. Strain the infusion and drink warm. Only drink one cup a day to support liver detox.

GAS AND BLOATING: CARMINATIVE HERBAL REMEDIES

Carminative herbs help ease bloating and gently relieve gas, keeping your digestion comfortable and stress-free.

CUMIN TEA

Stimulates digestion and reduces bloating.

Ingredients

- 1 cup hot water
- 1 tsp cumin seeds

Instructions

- In a small pot, bring cumin seeds and water to a boil for five minutes. Strain the liquid and drink warm.

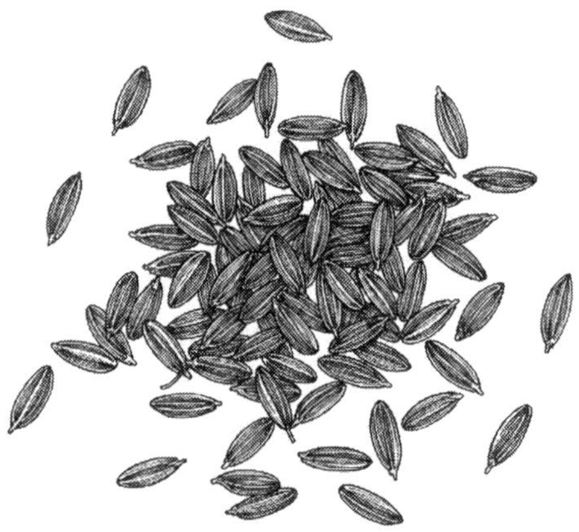

CHAMOMILE TEA

Relaxes the digestive tract and reduces gas.

Ingredients

- 1 cup hot water
- 1 tbsp dried chamomile flowers

Instructions

- Use hot water to steep the flowers for 10 minutes while covered. Strain and drink warm after meals.

HOLY BASIL (TULSI) TEA

Reduces gas and bloating while calming the digestive system.

Ingredients

- 1 cup hot water
- 1 tbsp dried or fresh holy basil leaves

Instructions

- Use hot water to steep the herb for 10 minutes while covered. Strain and drink warm to relieve bloating and promote digestion.

ORANGE PEEL TEA

Supports digestion and reduces bloating by stimulating digestive enzymes.

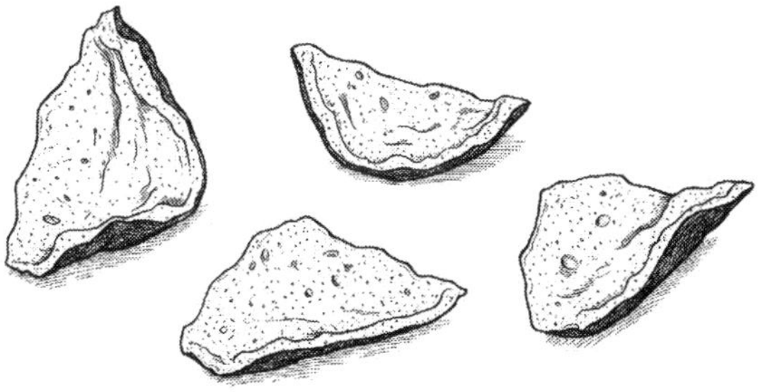

Ingredients

- 1 cup hot water
- 1 tbsp dried orange peel (organic)

Instructions

- Steep dried orange peel in hot water for 10 minutes. Strain and drink warm after meals to ease bloating and discomfort.

GUT FLORA IMBALANCE: HERBAL PREBIOTICS FOR A HEALTHY MICROBIOME

Nourishing your beneficial gut bacteria with herbal sources of prebiotics and resistant starch is a natural way to support a healthy, balanced microbiome.

TRIPHALA POWDER DRINK

Supports gut health and regularity.

Ingredients

- 1 cup warm water
- ½ tsp triphala powder

Instructions

- Stir triphala powder into warm water and drink before bedtime.

GARLIC INFUSION

Acts as a prebiotic to support beneficial gut bacteria.

Ingredients

- 1 cup warm water
- 1 clove garlic, crushed

Instructions

- Steep crushed garlic in warm water for 10 minutes. Strain and drink.

SPIRULINA DRINK

Rich in prebiotic compounds that support beneficial gut bacteria.

Ingredients

- 1 cup water or coconut water
- 1 tsp spirulina powder
- ½ tsp honey (optional)

Instructions

- Stir spirulina powder into water until fully dissolved. Drink once a day.

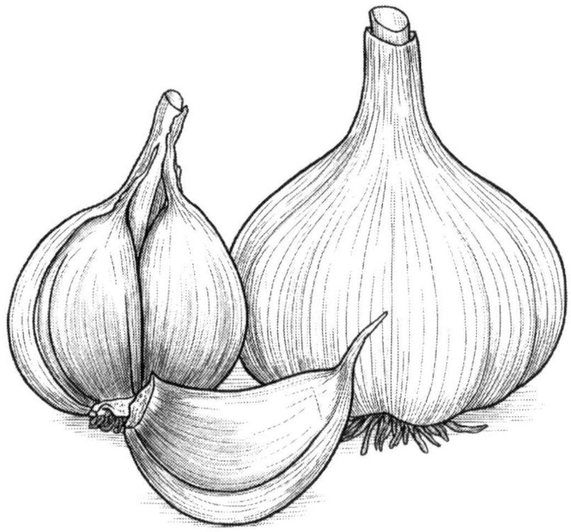

GREEN BANANA SMOOTHIE

High in resistant starch, which feeds beneficial gut bacteria.

Ingredients

- 1 green (unripe) banana
- 1 cup almond milk or water
- ½ tsp cinnamon (optional)

Instructions

- Peel and chop the green banana. Blend with almond milk or water until smooth. Add cinnamon if desired and drink fresh.

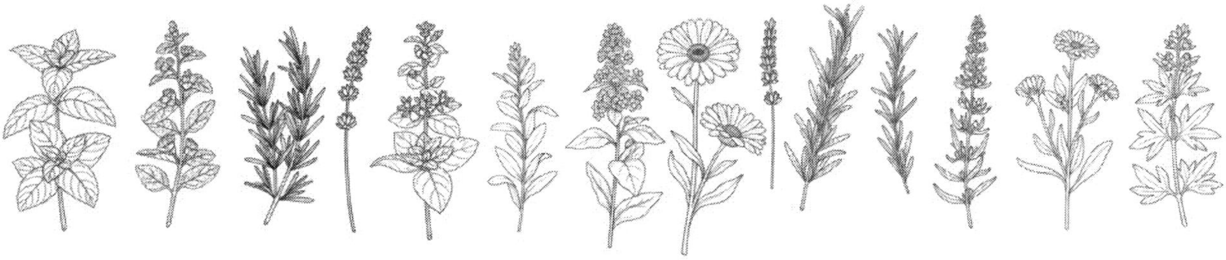

LIVER SUPPORT: HERBAL REMEDIES FOR LIVER DETOXIFICATION

These herbs help your liver function at its best, naturally supporting detoxification and overall wellness.

TURMERIC TEA

Reduces liver inflammation and supports detoxification.

Ingredients

- 2 cups water
- 1 tsp turmeric powder
- pinch of black pepper

Instructions

- Bring water, black pepper, and turmeric to a boil for 10 minutes. Strain and drink warm. Do not drink more than one cup a day.

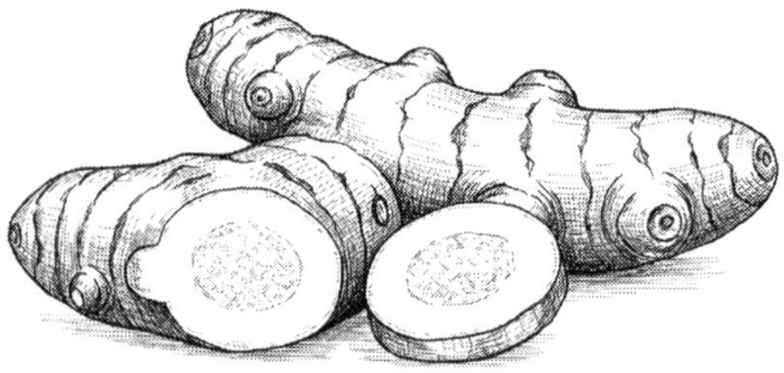

MILK THISTLE TEA

Protects liver cells and promotes regeneration.

Ingredients

- 1 cup hot water
- 1 tsp crushed milk thistle seeds

Instructions

- Use hot water to steep the seeds. Keep them covered for 10 minutes. Strain and drink warm once a day.

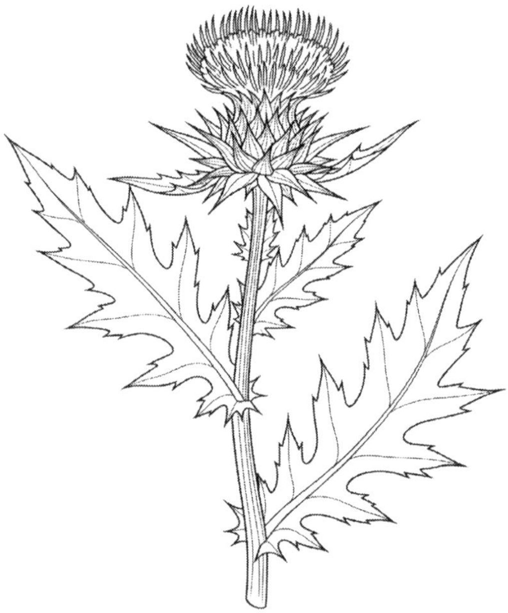

PARASITE CLEANSE: HERBAL REMEDIES TO ELIMINATE PARASITES

These herbs naturally help fight off parasites, giving your body extra support to stay clean and healthy.

WORMWOOD TEA

Helps expel parasites from the digestive system.

Ingredients

- 1 cup hot water
- ½ tsp dried wormwood leaves

Instructions

- Use hot water to steep the herb for five minutes while covered. Drink once a day for a maximum of two weeks.

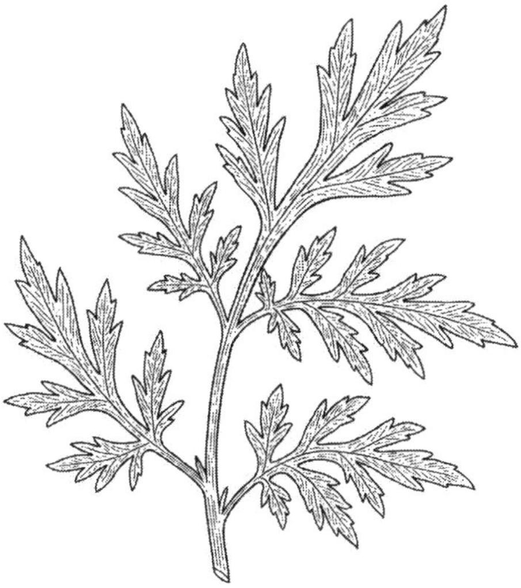

BLACK WALNUT HULL TEA

Acts as a natural antiparasitic agent.

Ingredients

- 2 cups water
- 1 tbsp dried black walnut hulls

Instructions

- Simmer black walnut hulls in water for 10 minutes. Strain and drink once daily.

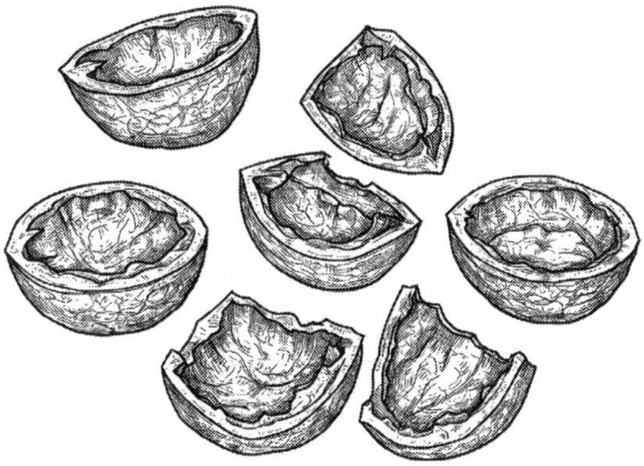

CHAPTER 8:

SKIN CARE AND WOUND HEALING

Herbs and natural remedies can do wonders for your skin, helping it heal and stay healthy. These simple, natural treatments work with your body's healing process, addressing skin concerns and boosting overall skin health along the way.

DRY SKIN: HERBAL MOISTURIZERS FOR HYDRATION

Natural moisturizers not only help to restore skin elasticity, but they can prevent the itchiness and dullness that is associated with dry skin.

SHEA BUTTER APPLICATION

Deeply hydrates and improves skin elasticity.

Ingredients

- 2 tbsp raw shea butter

Instructions

- Warm shea butter between your hands and massage into dry skin. Focus the application on areas that are prone to dryness, such as the elbows, knees, heels and hands.

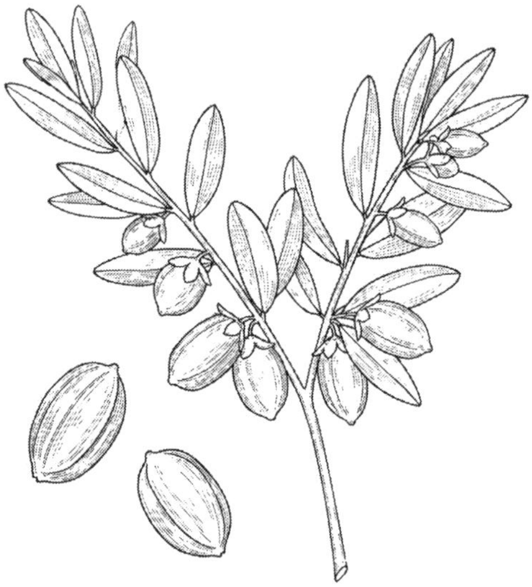

COCONUT OIL RUB

Softens and hydrates dry skin.

Ingredients

- 2 tbsp virgin coconut oil

Instructions

- Apply like a lotion. Allow it to absorb overnight. For best results, apply coconut oil on damp skin (such as after a bath or shower) to seal in moisture.

ARGAN OIL

A source of antioxidants and essential fatty acids; provides deep hydration.

Ingredients

- 3-4 drops of pure argan oil

Instructions

- Apply a few drops of argan oil to your palms. Massage gently onto your face or body. Use daily for a radiant, moisturized glow.

ALOE VERA GEL

Soothes and hydrates dry, irritated skin.

Ingredients

- 2 tbsp fresh aloe vera gel

Instructions

- Use like a lotion and apply to dry areas. Leave on for 15 minutes before rinsing or let it absorb naturally. It's suitable to use as a moisturizer for the face, especially for combination and oily skin types.

JOJOBA OIL

Balances skin moisture and mimics the skin's natural oils.

Ingredients

- 1–2 drops of pure jojoba oil

Instructions

- Apply a few drops of jojoba oil to your fingertips. Gently massage into the skin, focusing on dry areas. Use daily for soft, hydrated skin. The oil is suitable for all skin types and is safe to use on the face as it won't clog pores.

AVOCADO OIL

Rich in vitamins A, D, and E, helps nourish and hydrate dry skin.

Ingredients

- 1 tbsp avocado oil

Instructions

- Apply avocado oil to your skin after a shower or bath while your skin is still damp. Gently massage the oil into your skin for long-lasting hydration. Use as needed for smooth, nourished skin.

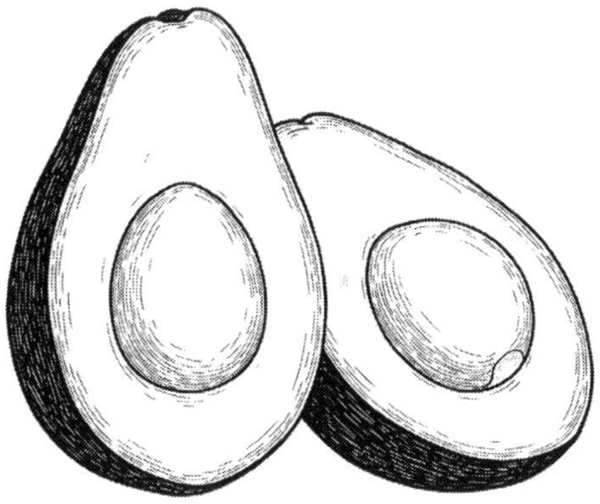

ACNE: HERBAL TREATMENTS FOR CLEAR SKIN

Herbs with antimicrobial and anti-inflammatory properties help reduce acne and prevent breakouts.

TEA TREE OIL SPOT TREATMENT

Fights acne-causing bacteria.

Ingredients

- 1 drop tea tree essential oil
- 1 tsp jojoba oil (carrier oil)

Instructions

- Mix tea tree oil with jojoba oil. Apply directly to blemishes with a cotton swab.

WITCH HAZEL ASTRINGENT

Tightens pores and reduces oiliness.

Ingredients

- 2 tbsp witch hazel extract
- ½ cup distilled water

Instructions

- Mix ingredients and store in a spray bottle. Use as a toner after cleansing.

GREEN TEA EXTRACT TONER

Reduces inflammation and sebum production.

Ingredients

- half a cup of cool green tea (already brewed)
- 1 tsp apple cider vinegar (optional)

Instructions

- Pour the ingredients into a small bottle and shake to combine. Apply with a cotton pad after cleansing.

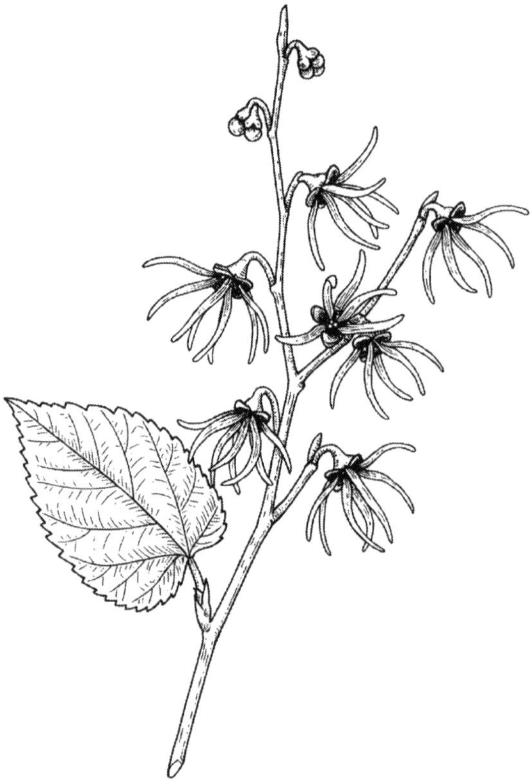

CALENDULA INFUSED OIL

Promotes skin healing and reduces redness.

Ingredients

- 1 cup of calendula flowers (dried or fresh)
- 1 cup of oil (olive, avocado, coconut, or grapeseed are good options)

Instructions

- Place the flowers in a glass jar and cover with oil. The flowers should be submerged. Place the lid on and allow the mixture to infuse in a warm, dark place for two weeks. After that, strain the oil into an amber container. To use, gently massage into clean, dry skin. Focus on areas with acne or irritation. Use daily for calming and healing properties.

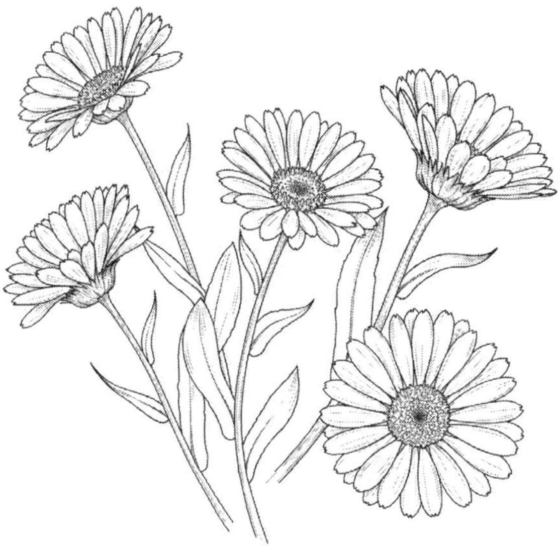

ALOE VERA AND TURMERIC FACE MASK

Reduces redness and fights acne-causing bacteria.

Ingredients

- 2 tbsp aloe vera gel
- 1 tsp turmeric powder

Instructions

- Mix aloe vera gel with turmeric powder to form a paste. Apply the mixture just like a mask. Take care to avoid sensitive areas around the eyes and mouth. Allow the mask to sit on your skin for 20 minutes, then gently rinse it off with warm water.

LAVENDER OIL SPOT TREATMENT

Reduces inflammation and promotes healing.

Ingredients

- 1 drop lavender essential oil
- 1 tsp aloe vera gel

Instructions

- Mix lavender oil with aloe vera gel. Use a cotton swab to apply to the affected areas. Leave on overnight for soothing acne relief.
-

MINOR CUTS AND SCRAPES: HERBAL ANTISEPTICS FOR WOUND CARE

These herbal remedies prevent infection and promote faster healing.

CALENDULA SALVE

Reduces inflammation and speeds wound healing.

Ingredients

- 1 tbsp dried calendula flowers
- ¼ cup coconut oil

Instructions

- Infuse calendula flowers in coconut oil over low heat for 20 minutes. Strain and store in a clean container. Apply to wounds as needed.

TURMERIC PASTE

Reduces inflammation and fights bacteria.

Ingredients

- 1 tsp turmeric powder
- 1 tsp water

Instructions

- Mix turmeric and water to form a paste. Apply to minor wounds and leave for 15 minutes before rinsing.

HONEY APPLICATION

Naturally antibacterial and promotes healing.

Ingredients

- 1 tsp raw honey

Instructions

- Apply a thin layer of honey to a minor cut or burn. Cover with a bandage.

GOLDENSEAL POWDER PASTE

Antibacterial and helps prevent infection.

Ingredients

- 1 tsp goldenseal powder
- 1 tsp water

Instructions

- Make a paste with the ingredients. Apply directly to the cut and let it sit for 15–20 minutes before rinsing. Repeat twice daily as needed.

ROSEMARY RINSE

Reduces inflammation and disinfects wounds.

Ingredients

- 1 cup hot water
- 1 tbsp dried or fresh rosemary leaves

Instructions

- Infuse the herb with hot water for 15 minutes. Let the infusion cool and use it to rinse cuts and scrapes. Repeat as needed.

ALOE AND TEA TREE GEL

Soothes wounds and fights bacteria.

Ingredients

- 1 tbsp aloe vera gel
- 2 drops tea tree essential oil

Instructions

- Combine the ingredients and apply as a thin layer on the wound. Repeat the treatment three times a day.

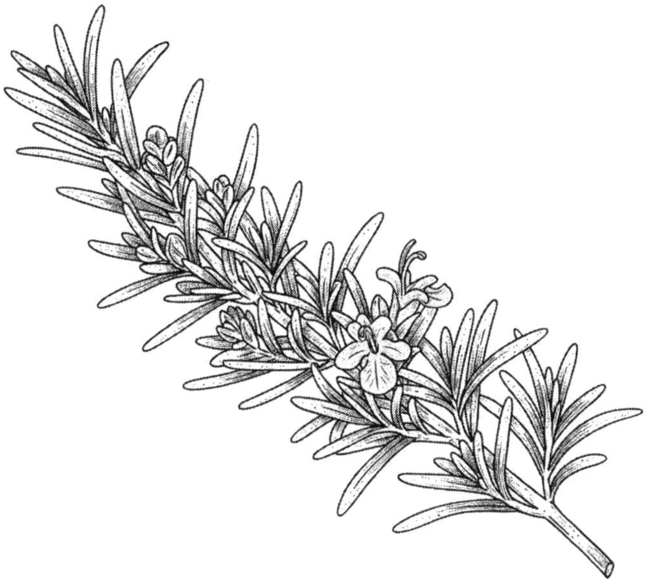

BURNS: HERBAL REMEDIES FOR SOOTHING RELIEF

These treatments help relieve pain and reduce inflammation from minor burns.

ALOE VERA GEL

Cools and heals burned skin.

Ingredients

- 2 tbsp fresh aloe vera gel

Instructions

- Gently apply a small blob of the aloe vera gel to any burned areas. Repeat up to three times daily.

LAVENDER ESSENTIAL OIL COMPRESS

Reduces pain and prevents infection.

Ingredients

- 3 drops lavender essential oil
- ½ cup cool water

Instructions

- Mix lavender oil with cool water. Soak a cloth in the mixture and apply to burns for 10 minutes.

HONEY BURN APPLICATION

Soothes pain and promotes healing.

Ingredients

- 1 tsp raw honey

Instructions

- In a thin layer, apply honey directly to the burn. Allow the honey to sit on the burn site for 20 minutes, then rinse off. Reapply up to three times a day. For severe burns, it is best to get help from a medical professional. If the burn does not show visible improvement within three days or is starting to show signs of infection (redness, swelling, smelling bad), it is strongly advised to seek immediate medical attention.

CHAMOMILE TEA RINSE

Calms inflammation and speeds healing.

Ingredients

- 1 cup hot water
- 1 tbsp dried chamomile flowers

Instructions

- Infuse the herb into hot water for 10 minutes while covered. Let the tea cool completely, then gently pour over the burn or soak a cloth in the tea and apply as a compress. For larger burn sites, make a strong infusion of chamomile and pour into a cool bath. Soak in the bath for 20 minutes, then gently pat the site dry and moisturize with aloe vera gel.

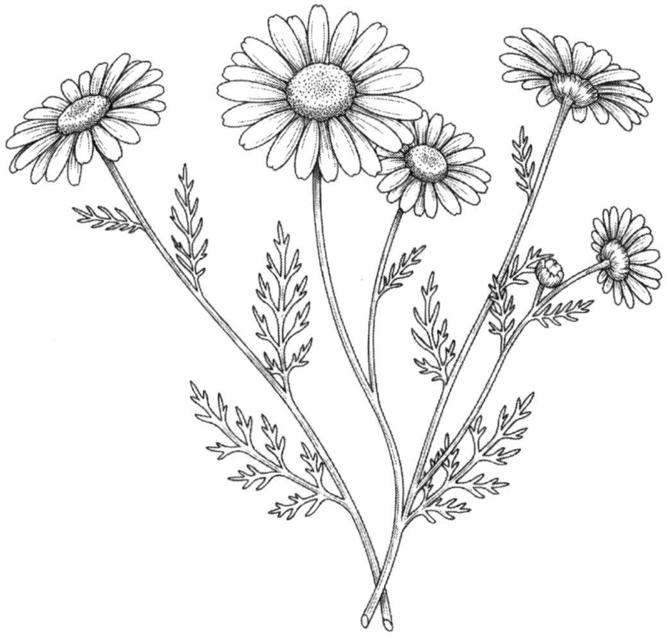

ECZEMA AND PSORIASIS: HERBAL SOAKS FOR INFLAMMATION REDUCTION

Herbal baths soothe irritated skin and relieve itching.

OATMEAL BATH

Moisturizes and calms inflamed skin. Colloidal oatmeal is a finely ground form of oatmeal that absorbs water.

Ingredients

- 1 cup colloidal oatmeal

Instructions

- Add oatmeal to a warm bath. The bathwater should be milky in color and silky to the touch. Soak for 20 minutes. This remedy is gentle enough to use with every bath. For best results, apply virgin coconut oil to damp skin after the bath to lock in moisture.

CHAMOMILE INFUSION BATH

Reduces itching and inflammation.

Ingredients

- 2 tbsp dried chamomile flowers
- 2 cups boiling water

Instructions

- Use boiling water and steep the flowers for 15 minutes while covered. Strain and add to the bathwater. Use this remedy at night and moisturize damp skin with coconut oil after the bath.

NEEM LEAF BATH

Soothes irritation and has antimicrobial properties.

Ingredients

- ½ cup dried neem leaves
- 2 cups boiling water

Instructions

- Steep neem leaves in boiling water for 15 minutes. Strain and add the infusion to the bathwater. Soak for 20 minutes. Complete the treatment with coconut oil as a moisturizer.

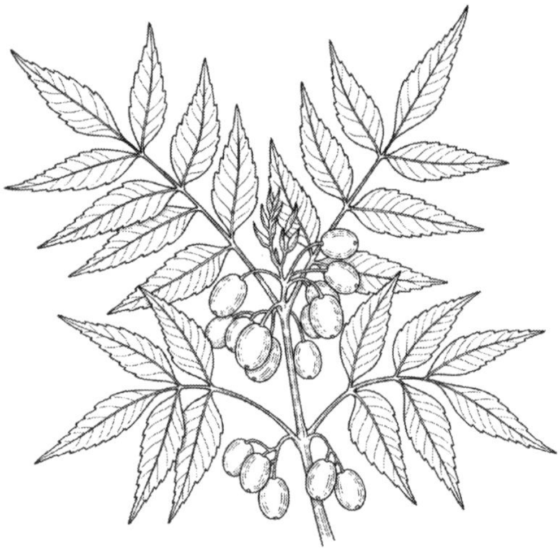

LAVENDER AND EPSOM SALT BATH

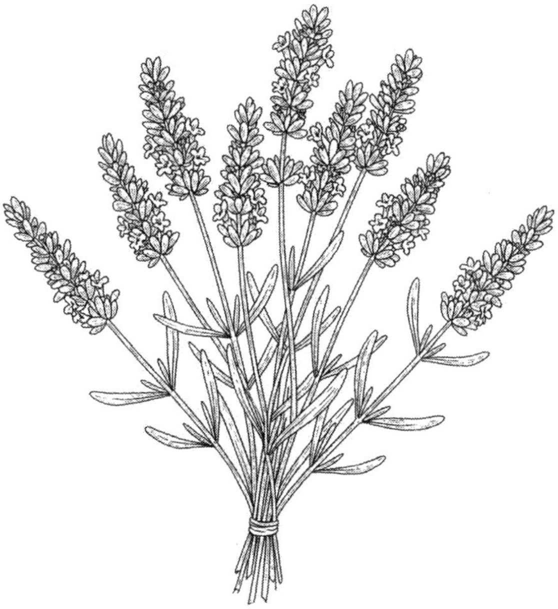

Reduces inflammation and promotes skin healing.

Ingredients

- ½ cup Epsom salt
- 10 drops of lavender essential oil

Instructions

- To a warm bath, add the essential oil and Epsom salt. Ensure the ingredients are dissolved. Soak for 20 minutes.

SCARS: HERBAL APPLICATIONS FOR SCAR REDUCTION

Some herbs can actually help your skin heal and fade scars, making them less noticeable over time. With consistent use, they can support natural regeneration and leave your skin looking smoother and healthier.

ROSEHIP SEED OIL MASSAGE

Improves skin texture and reduces discoloration.

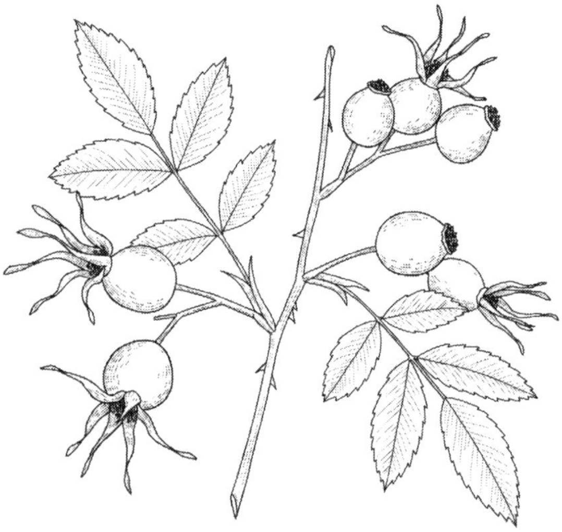

Ingredients

- 1 tsp rosehip seed oil

Instructions

- Massage oil into scars twice daily. Use small circular movements to massage the oil into the scar site.

GOTU KOLA EXTRACT APPLICATION

Enhances skin repair and improves elasticity.

Ingredients

- 1 tsp gotu kola extract

Instructions

- Apply the extract to scars daily.

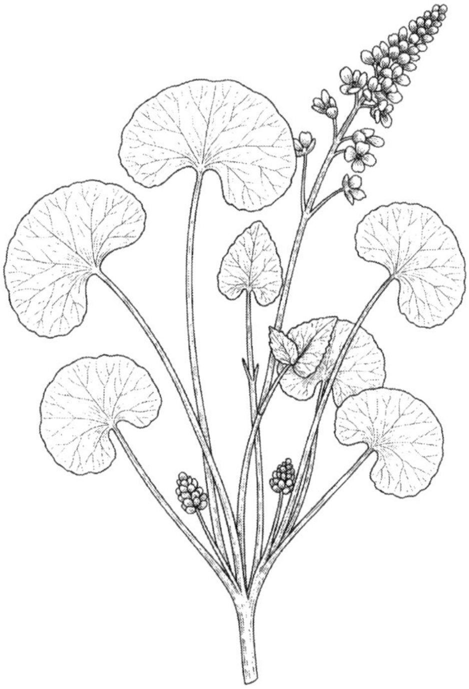

CALENDULA INFUSED OIL

Promotes skin regeneration and reduces scar visibility.

- See *Acne: Herbal Treatments for Clear Skin* for detailed instructions to make the oil. Massage the oil onto scars in small circular motions twice a day to reduce their appearance.

ALOE VERA AND VITAMIN E GEL

Hydrates the skin and improves scar healing.

Ingredients

- 2 tbsp fresh aloe vera gel
- 1 capsule of vitamin E oil

Instructions

- Mix aloe vera gel with the contents of a vitamin E capsule. Apply to scars and let it absorb into the skin. Use twice daily.

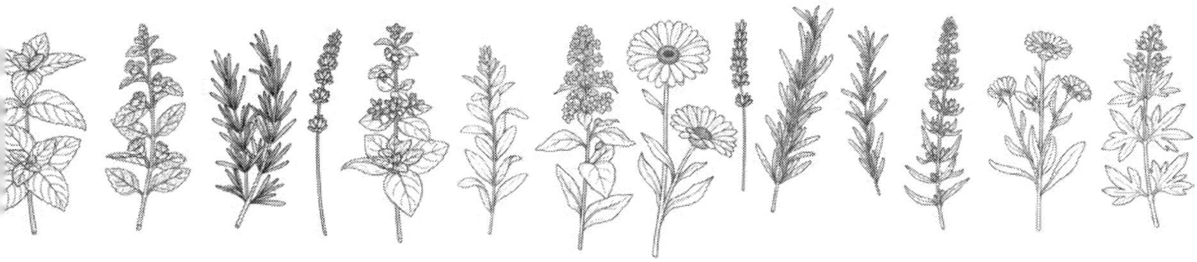

INSECT BITES AND STINGS: HERBAL REMEDIES FOR ITCH RELIEF

These remedies soothe irritation and reduce swelling.

BASIL LEAF RUB

Provides natural anti-itch benefits.

Ingredients

- fresh basil leaves

Instructions

- Crush basil leaves to form a paste and apply to the bite. Allow the leaf paste to sit on the bite site for 10 - 20 minutes, then rinse off with lukewarm water.

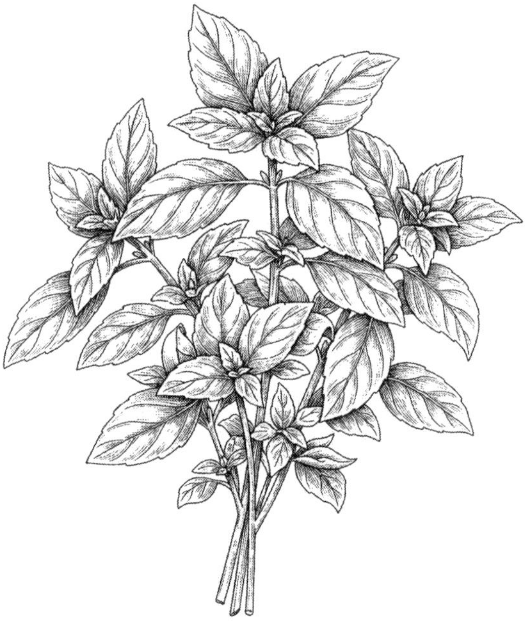

ALOE VERA AND PEPPERMINT GEL

Soothes irritation and provides a cooling effect.

Ingredients

- 1 tbsp fresh aloe vera gel
- 1 drop peppermint essential oil

Instructions

- Combine the ingredients in a small container. Apply a thin layer to the bite. Reapply as needed to reduce itching and inflammation.

LAVENDER ESSENTIAL OIL APPLICATION

Soothes irritation and promotes healing.

Ingredients

- 1 drop lavender essential oil
- 1 tsp coconut oil (carrier oil)

Instructions

Combine the ingredients and apply as needed to the bite site.

PLANTAIN LEAF POULTICE

Draws out toxins and reduces inflammation.

Ingredients

- 2 fresh plantain leaves

Instructions

- Create a paste by crushing the leaves. Then apply to the affected area and allow the poultice to sit for 20 minutes.

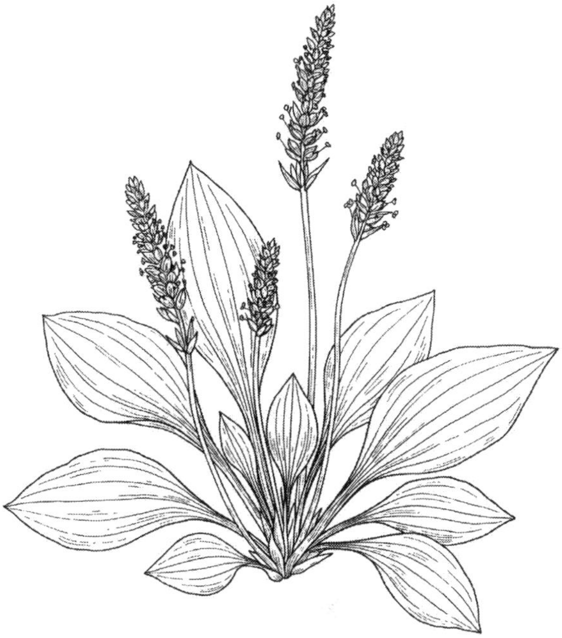

FUNGAL INFECTIONS: HERBAL ANTIFUNGAL TREATMENTS

Dealing with athlete's foot or ringworm? Some natural remedies can help soothe irritation and speed up healing.

GARLIC PASTE

Contains powerful antifungal properties.

Ingredients

- 2 garlic cloves, crushed

Instructions

- Apply crushed garlic to the affected area. Leave for 10 minutes, then rinse.

APPLE CIDER VINEGAR SOAK

Balances skin pH and fights fungal infections.

Ingredients

- ½ cup apple cider vinegar
- 2 cups warm water

Instructions

- Combine the ingredients and soak the affected area for 15 minutes. Repeat this treatment twice a day.

TEA TREE OIL APPLICATION

Inhibits fungal growth.

Ingredients

- 2 drops tea tree oil
- 1 tsp coconut oil (carrier oil)

Instructions

- Mix oils and apply to the infection twice daily.

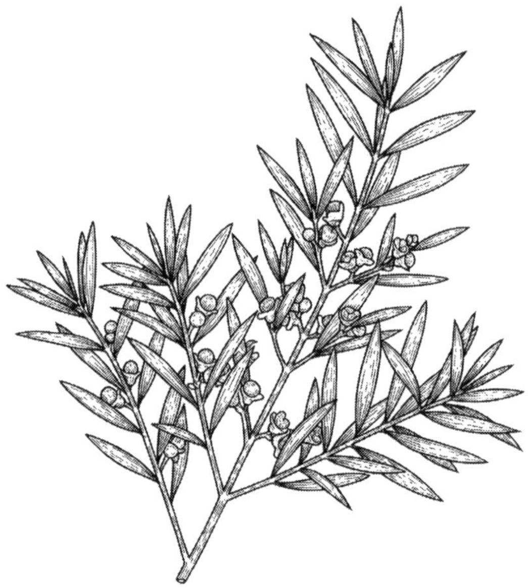

TURMERIC PASTE

Reduces inflammation and combats fungal infections.

Ingredients

- 1 tsp turmeric powder
- 1 tsp water or coconut oil

Instructions

- Combine the ingredients to create a paste. Apply and allow to sit on the affected area for 20 minutes. Rinse and repeat once daily.

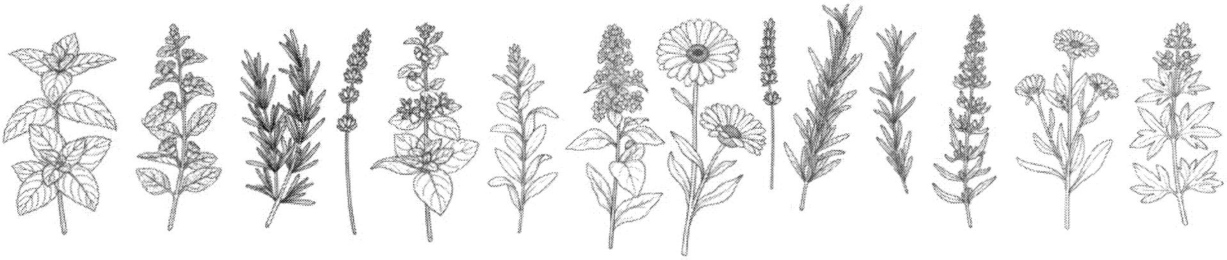

SUNBURN: HERBAL REMEDIES FOR RECOVERY

Burned skin can be soothed naturally with herbs and remedies that ease discomfort and reduce redness, helping your skin heal faster.

CUCUMBER SLICES

Reduces swelling and hydrates sunburned skin.

Ingredients

- ½ cucumber, sliced

Instructions

- Place cool cucumber slices on the affected areas. For larger sunburnt areas, blend the cucumber until smooth. Then soak a clean muslin cloth in the juice and apply to the affected areas for 20 minutes. Thereafter, gently remove the cloth and rinse off any residue with cool water.

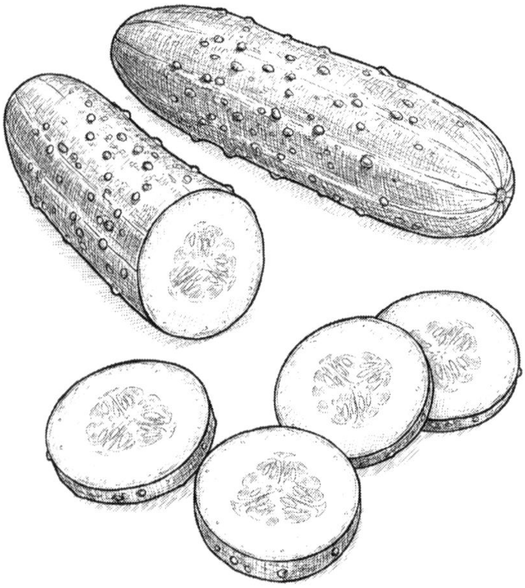

PEPPERMINT TEA SPRAY

Provides a cooling effect on sunburned skin.

Ingredients

- 1 cup brewed peppermint tea, cooled

Instructions

- Pour tea into a spray bottle. Spritz onto sunburned skin as needed.

ALOE AND COCONUT OIL LOTION

Deeply hydrates and soothes sunburned skin.

Ingredients

- 2 tbsp fresh aloe vera gel
- 1 tbsp coconut oil

Instructions

Mix aloe vera gel and coconut oil until well combined. Apply gently to sunburned skin. Repeat three times daily for relief. For best results, combine with an oatmeal bath.

OATMEAL BATH

Reduces redness and soothes irritation.

See *Eczema and Psoriasis: Herbal Soaks for Inflammation Reduction* for detailed instructions. Moisturize with aloe and coconut oil lotion for best results.

CHAPTER 9:

PAIN AND INFLAMMATION RELIEF

Got a headache, sore muscles, or creaky joints? Herbal and natural remedies can help ease pain and inflammation while giving your body the boost it needs to heal itself – no harsh chemicals required. The natural remedies in this chapter are easy to prepare and administer while being gentle on the body.

HEADACHES AND MIGRAINES: HERBAL REMEDIES FOR RELIEF

Some herbs are like nature's aspirin – they can help to soothe headache pain and calm inflammation at the same time.

FEVERFEW TEA

Reduces migraine frequency and severity.

Ingredients

- 1 tsp dried feverfew leaves
- 1 cup hot water

Instructions

- Steep the ingredients for 10 minutes while covered. Strain and drink once daily.

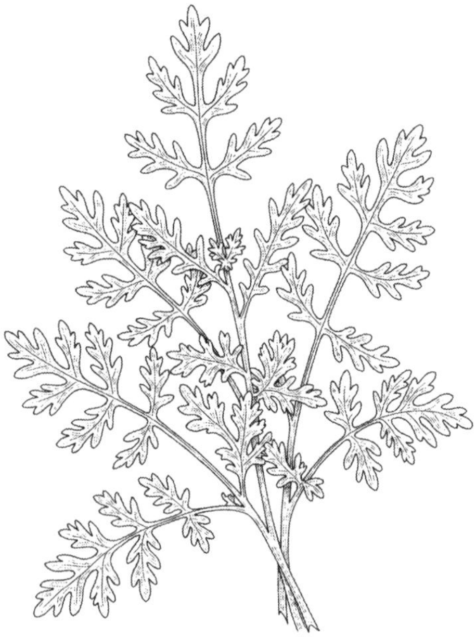

PEPPERMINT OIL APPLICATION

Relieves tension headaches and improves circulation.

Ingredients

- 2 drops peppermint essential oil
- 1 tsp coconut oil (carrier oil)

Instructions

- Mix oils and apply to temples. Gently massage in circular motions.

WILLOW BARK TEA

Provides pain relief similar to aspirin.

Ingredients

- 1 tsp dried willow bark
- 1 cup hot water

Instructions

- Steep willow bark in hot water for 15 minutes. Strain and drink up to twice daily. Avoid use if you're sensitive to aspirin.

LAVENDER STEAM INHALATION

Eases stress-related headaches and promotes relaxation.

Ingredients

- 3 drops lavender essential oil
- 1 bowl hot water

Instructions

- Pour piping hot water into a vessel or a wide bowl. Use a towel to trap the steam as you lean over to inhale the calming vapors for 10 minutes. Do this at night, before bedtime, for best results..

BASIL TEA

Relaxes muscles and helps relieve headaches caused by tension.

Ingredients

- 1 tsp dried basil leaves (or 3 fresh leaves)
- 1 cup hot water

Instructions

- Steep basil in hot water for 10 minutes. Strain and sip slowly while inhaling the calming aroma.

ROSEMARY SCALP MASSAGE

Improves circulation and helps relieve tension headaches.

Ingredients

- 3 drops rosemary essential oil
- 1 tsp carrier oil (olive, coconut, avocado, or jojoba works well)

Instructions

- Mix the oils and massage them into your scalp for five minutes. Let it sit for a few minutes and inhale the calming scent deeply before rinsing. Alternatively, you can leave it in for extended relief. As a bonus, rosemary essential oil nourishes the hair follicles, simulating hair growth, so choose a carrier oil that your scalp loves.

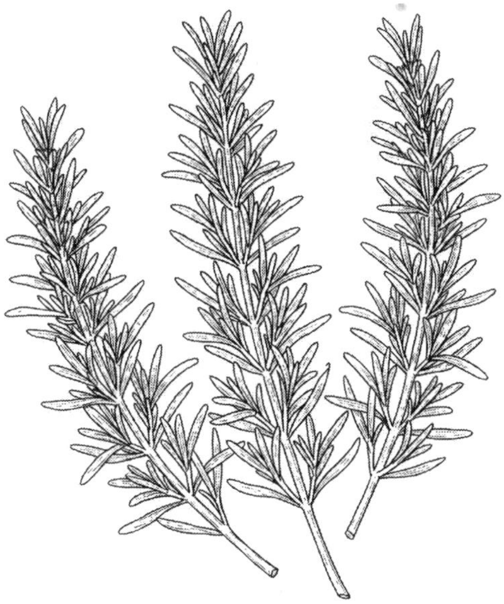

MUSCLE PAIN: HERBAL COMPRESSES AND SALVES

Post-exercise inflammation can be a painful ordeal; luckily nature's pharmacy has gentle and effective cures on hand to soothe sore muscles.

GINGER COMPRESS

Improves circulation and relieves muscle pain.

Ingredients

- 2 tbsp grated fresh ginger
- 1 cloth

Instructions

- Wrap ginger in a cloth and soak in warm water. Apply to sore muscles for 15 minutes.

TURMERIC PASTE

Reduces inflammation and pain.

Ingredients

- 1 tbsp turmeric powder
- 2 tbsp warm water

Instructions

- Make a paste with the ingredients and apply to sore muscles. Allow the remedy to sit for 20 minutes before rinsing off.

HOMEMADE TIGER BALM

Relieves muscle pain, stiffness, and improves circulation.

Ingredients

- 5 drops cinnamon essential oil
- 10 drops wintergreen essential oil
- 1 tbsp camphor essential oil
- 10 drops eucalyptus essential oil
- 2 tbsp coconut oil
- 2 tbsp beeswax
- 10 drops peppermint essential oil

Instructions

- Melt beeswax and coconut oil together in a double boiler until fully combined. Remove from heat, carefully stir in the essential oils, and pour into containers. Once cooled, it's ready to apply to sore muscles for relief.

ARNICA SALVE

Reduces swelling and muscle soreness.

Ingredients

- 2 tbsp arnica-infused oil
- 1 tbsp beeswax

Instructions

- To make the infused oil, you need to place dried arnica flowers in a clean glass jar. Then, submerge the flowers in olive oil. Seal the jar tightly and place it in a warm spot for three weeks to infuse. Alternatively, you can use a double boiler to gently heat the oil and arnica flowers over low heat for two hours. When the oil is ready, strain into an amber container. Use the infused oil and combine with melted beeswax to create a salve. Use the salve as needed to bring relief to sore muscles.

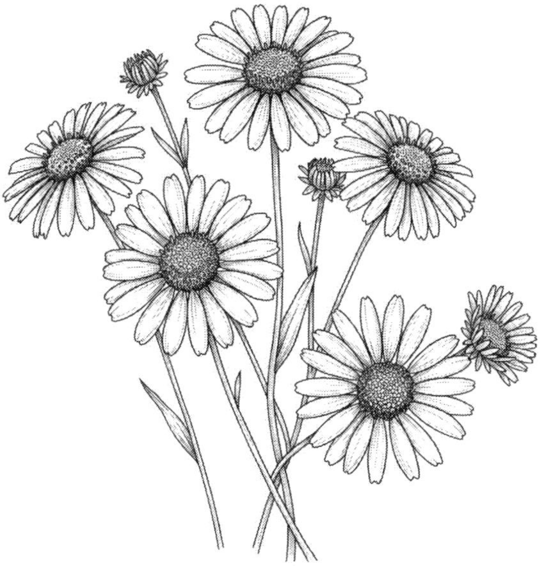

CAYENNE SALVE

Warms muscles and helps relieve deep-seated pain.

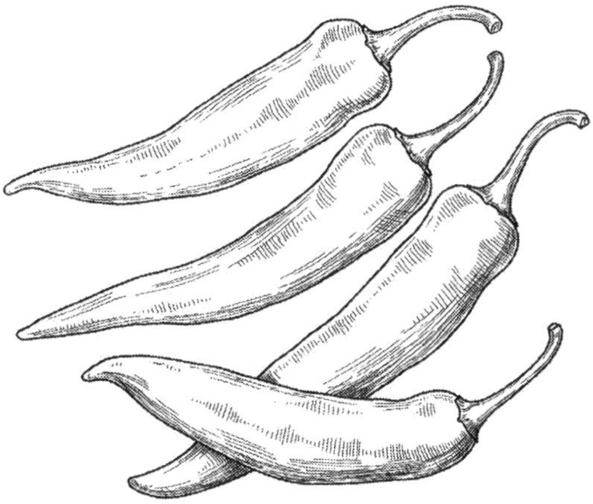

Ingredients

- 1 tsp cayenne pepper powder
- 2 tbsp olive oil
- 1 tbsp beeswax

Instructions

- Melt beeswax and mix with cayenne and olive oil. Let cool and apply a small amount to sore muscles. Avoid contact with the eyes or broken skin.

COMFREY POULTICE

Promotes healing and eases muscle pain.

Ingredients

- 1 tbsp dried comfrey leaves
- 2 tbsp warm water
- 1 cloth

Instructions

- Mix comfrey with warm water to create a paste. Spread onto a cloth and apply to sore muscles for 20 minutes.

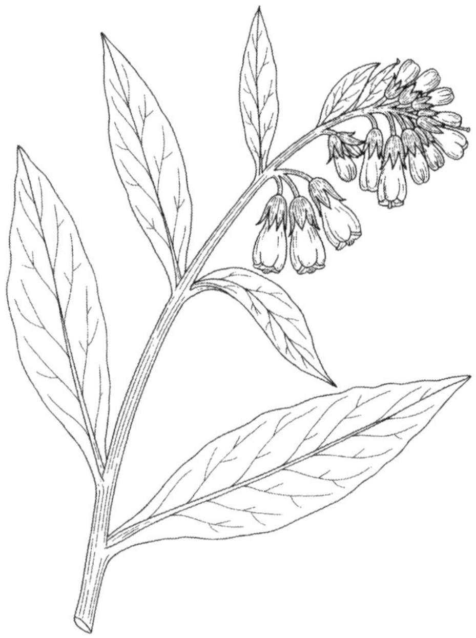

EPSOM SALT AND LAVENDER BATH SOAK

Relaxes muscles and soothes inflammation.

Ingredients

- 1 cup Epsom salt
- 1 tbsp dried lavender flowers
- 5 drops lavender essential oil

Instructions

Add ingredients to warm bathwater. Soak for 15–20 minutes to alleviate sore muscles. This remedy is best done at night, before bedtime.

PEPPERMINT AND WINTERGREEN MASSAGE OIL

Provides a cooling effect and helps relax tense muscles.

Ingredients

- 3 drops peppermint essential oil
- 3 drops wintergreen essential oil
- 1 tsp carrier oil (coconut, olive, avocado or jojoba)

Instructions

- Mix the oils and massage into sore muscles using circular motions. Allow the oil to absorb for lasting relief.

JOINT PAIN: HERBAL REMEDIES FOR ARTHRITIS RELIEF

Joint pain, especially from arthritis, can often feel like it puts your life on hold, but there is hope. A diet rich in Omega-3s and targeted herbal treatments can bring relief from the debilitating pain.

BOSWELLIA OIL MASSAGE

Improves mobility and reduces swelling. The Biblical incense frankincense is an extract from the resin of the Boswellia sacra tree, and essential oils and extracts are readily available.

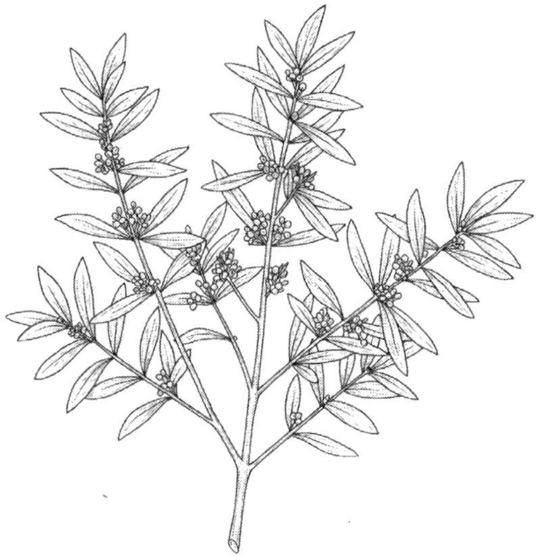

Ingredients

- 5 drops boswellia essential oil
- 1 tbsp coconut or olive oil

Instructions

- Mix oils and massage into affected joints twice daily.

DEVIL'S CLAW TEA

Relieves arthritis and chronic joint pain.

Ingredients

- 1 tsp dried devil's claw root
- 1 cup hot water

Instructions

- Use hot water and steep the herb (covered) for 15 minutes. Strain and drink once a day..

EUCALYPTUS OIL APPLICATION

Cools inflammation and eases discomfort.

Ingredients

- 3 drops eucalyptus essential oil
- 1 tbsp carrier oil

Instructions

- Mix the oils and massage into painful joints. Use as often as needed.

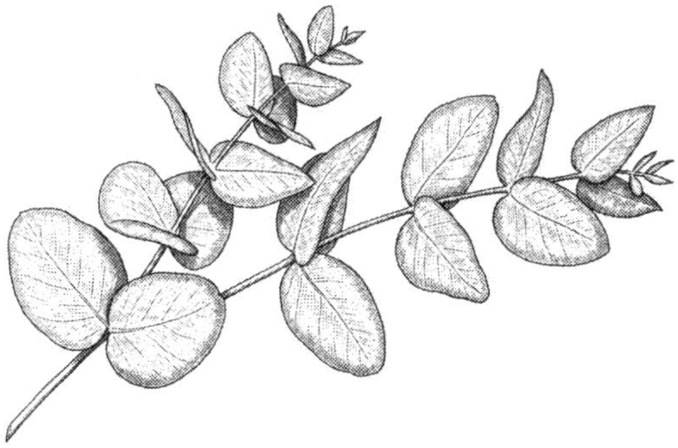

ASHWAGANDHA MILK

Reduces inflammation, boosts strength, and helps with joint stiffness.

Ingredients

- 1 tsp Ashwagandha powder
- 1 cup warm milk
- Honey (optional)

Instructions

- Mix the Ashwagandha powder into warm milk. Stir well and drink once a day before bed to reduce inflammation and promote relaxation. You can add honey to enhance the taste and improve the soothing effect.

TURMERIC AND GHEE PASTE

Reduces joint pain and inflammation through its natural anti-inflammatory properties.

Ingredients

- 1 tbsp turmeric powder
- 1 tbsp ghee (clarified butter)

Instructions

- Mix the turmeric powder with warm ghee to create a paste. Apply the paste directly to the affected joint. Leave it on for 20–30 minutes before washing off with lukewarm water. Do this three times a week for relief.

GOLDEN MILK

Reduces inflammation and alleviates joint pain.

Ingredients

- 1 cup milk (or non-dairy milk like almond or coconut)
- 1 tsp turmeric powder
- 1/2 tsp cinnamon powder
- 1/4 tsp black pepper
- 1 tsp honey
- 1 tsp coconut oil or ghee (optional, but helps absorption)

Instructions

- Heat milk until it is steaming (but not boiling). Stir in turmeric, cinnamon, black pepper, and coconut oil or ghee. Simmer for 5–10 minutes, stirring occasionally. Remove from heat, strain, and sweeten with honey. Drink once a day to help reduce inflammation and support joint health.

MENSTRUAL CRAMPS: HERBAL TEAS FOR RELIEF

These simple and tasty teas can help relax the uterine muscles and ease menstrual cramps, providing natural relief during your period.

CINNAMON TEA

Improves circulation and reduces discomfort.

Ingredients

- 1 cinnamon stick
- 1 cup hot water

Instructions

- Steep cinnamon in hot water for 10 minutes. Remove the cinnamon stick and sweeten with honey if desired. Drink twice daily.

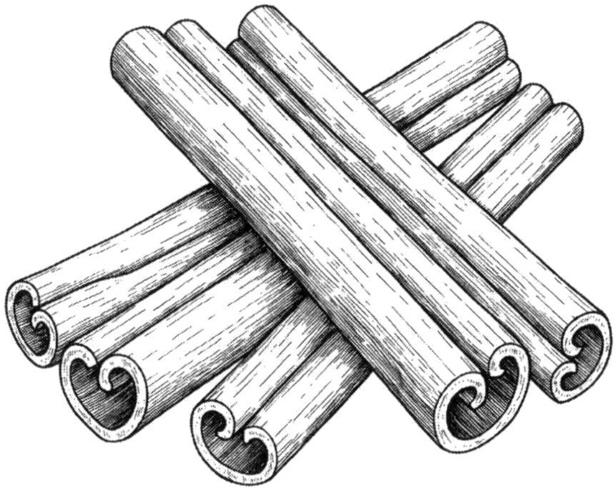

CHAMOMILE TEA

Eases menstrual pain and relaxes muscles.

For detailed brewing instructions, see Chapter Seven, *Gas and Bloating: Carminative Herbal Remedies.*

GINGER TEA

Reduces inflammation and soothes cramps.

For detailed brewing instructions, see Chapter Six, *Cold and Flu: Herbal Teas for Symptom Relief..*

TOOTHACHE: HERBAL PAIN RELIEVERS

Natural remedies with antibacterial and numbing properties can be a real lifesaver when you're dealing with tooth pain and gum discomfort.

CLOVE OIL APPLICATION

Numbs pain and fights bacteria. In some historic cases patients were recommended to chew directly on cloves, however using essential oil makes the treatment easier.

Ingredients

- 1 drop clove essential oil
- 1 cotton ball

Instructions

- Soak cotton ball in clove oil and place it on the affected tooth.

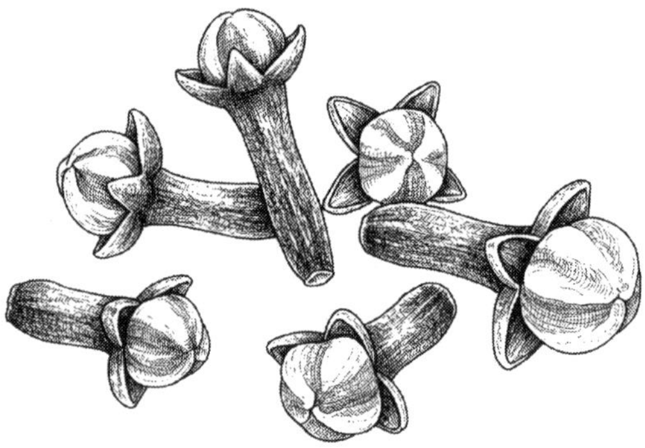

PEPPERMINT TEA RINSE

Provides natural pain relief.

Ingredients

- 1 cup brewed peppermint tea

Instructions

- Use cooled tea as a mouth rinse. See Chapter Six, *Cold and Flu: Herbal Teas for Symptom Relief*, for detailed brewing instructions.

GARLIC PASTE

Acts as a natural antimicrobial.

Ingredients

- 1 clove garlic, crushed

Instructions

- Apply crushed garlic to the affected tooth for 5–10 minutes.

CLOVE AND SALT MOUTHWASH

Numbs tooth pain and eases gum discomfort while fighting the bacteria that causes bad breath.

Ingredients

- 1 tsp ground cloves
- 1 tsp sea salt
- 1 cup hot water

Instructions

- To a cup, add the ground cloves and sea salt. Pour hot water over and cover the cup. Allow the mixture to infuse until cooled. Then strain and use as a mouthwash and gargle. Do not swallow.

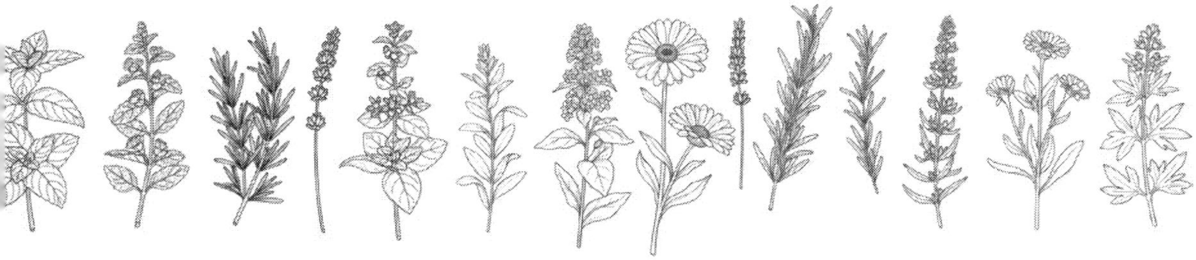

BACK PAIN: HERBAL APPLICATIONS FOR RELIEF

Tense muscles and a painful lower back can steal your quality of life, making even the simplest tasks, like bending down to pick something up, feel impossible. But the good news is, simple natural remedies can step in and help you reclaim your life, easing the pain and bringing back your freedom.

CAPSAICIN CREAM

Blocks pain signals.

Ingredients

- ½ tsp cayenne pepper
- 2 tbsp coconut oil

Instructions

- Mix and apply to sore areas as needed for relief from pain and stiffness.

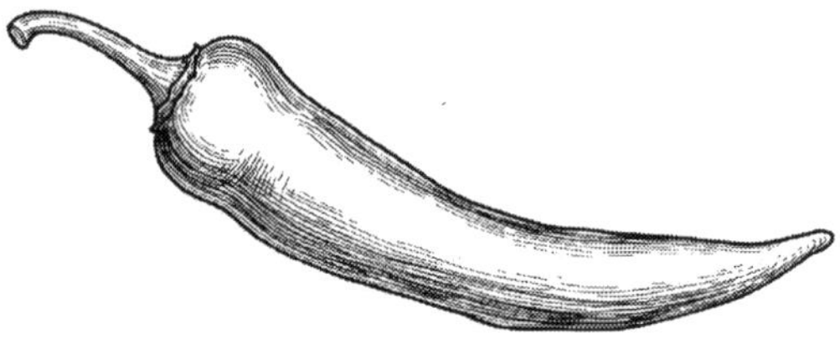

WILLOW BARK INFUSION

Acts as a natural anti-inflammatory.

Ingredients

- 1 tsp dried willow bark
- 1 cup hot water

Instructions

- Steep the herb (covered) in hot water for 15 minutes. Drink up to twice daily.

LAVENDER OIL BATH

Relaxes muscles and relieves pain.

Ingredients

- 5-10 drops of lavender essential oil

Instructions

- Add oil to warm bathwater and soak for 20 minutes. This remedy is best at night before bedtime.

MUSTARD SEED PLASTER

Increases blood flow and warms sore muscles, reducing stiffness.

Ingredients

- 2 tbsp mustard seed powder
- 2 tbsp warm water
- 1 thin cloth or gauze

Instructions

- Mix mustard seed powder with warm water to form a paste. Spread the paste onto a thin cloth. Place the cloth over the painful area. Leave on for 10–15 minutes, then remove and rinse.
-

FENUGREEK SEED PASTE

Reduces inflammation and provides deep muscle relaxation.

Ingredients

- 2 tbsp fenugreek seeds
- Warm water (enough to form a paste)

Instructions

- Grind the seeds to create a powder. Add warm water slowly to form a thick paste. Apply to the sore area and leave for 20 minutes before rinsing off. Repeat once daily for relief.

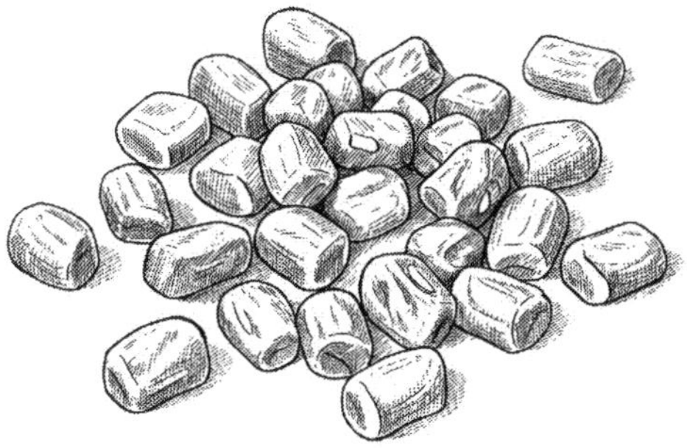

CLOVE AND BLACK SEED OIL RUB

Provides deep pain relief and improves circulation.

Ingredients

- 1 tbsp black seed oil
- 3 drops clove essential oil

Instructions

- Mix the oils together and massage into sore areas twice daily for relief.

NERVE PAIN: HERBAL REMEDIES FOR NEUROPATHIC RELIEF

Neuropathic pain can feel like an unrelenting burn, sharp shooting sensations, or numbness, making everyday activities a struggle. It happens when nerves get damaged or misfire, sending pain signals to the brain even when there's no injury. While it can be tough to manage, there are natural remedies that can help soothe this kind of pain, reduce inflammation, and improve nerve function, offering some much-needed relief.

ST. JOHN'S WORT TEA

Soothes nerve pain and inflammation.

Ingredients

- 1 tsp dried St. John's Wort
- 1 cup hot water

Instructions

- Steep in hot water for 10 minutes. Strain and drink daily.

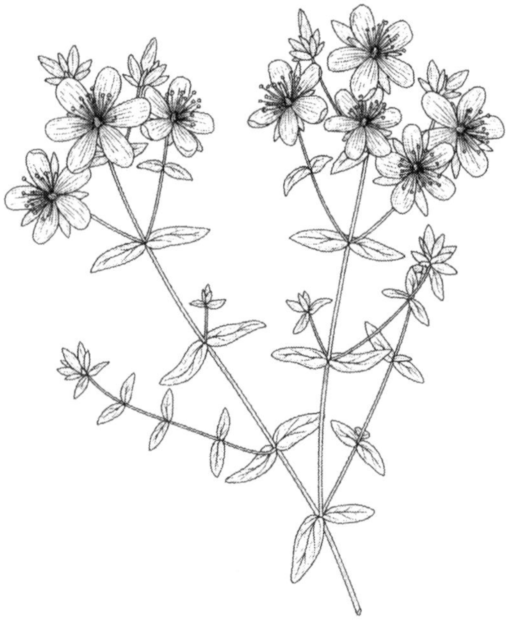

SKULLCAP TINCTURE

Helps calm the nervous system and ease nerve pain.

Ingredients

- 1 cup dried skullcap herb
- 2 cups alcohol (such as vodka or brandy)

Instructions

- Place the dried skullcap in your jar, pour the alcohol over the herbs, ensuring they're completely covered. Seal and store for six weeks in a cupboard that's cool and dark.. Afterwards, strain out the herbs using a fine-mesh strainer or cheesecloth, and transfer the liquid into a clean bottle or dropper bottle for easy use. To use, take 20-30 drops of the tincture in a small amount of water, once or twice a day, to help soothe nerve pain.

SYSTEMIC INFLAMMATION: HERBAL TEAS FOR FULL-BODY RELIEF

Systemic inflammation often goes unnoticed until it causes discomfort or even chronic conditions. It happens when the immune system becomes overactive and starts attacking healthy tissues, leading to pain, fatigue, and other symptoms. Managing systemic inflammation is key to feeling better, and natural remedies can help calm the immune response, reduce inflammation, and restore balance to the body, offering relief from the inside out.

GREEN TEA

Contains powerful antioxidants.

For detailed brewing instructions, see Chapter Seven, *Leaky Gut Syndrome: Herbal Remedies for Gut Lining Repair.*

GOTU KOLA AND GINGER TEA

Supports inflammation reduction and promotes circulation.

Ingredients

- 1 tsp dried Gotu Kola leaves
- 1 inch fresh ginger root, sliced
- 1 cup hot water

Instructions

- Use a small pot and bring the ginger slices and water to a boil for 7 minutes. Add Gotu Kola and steep for another 5 minutes. Strain, then drink to help reduce inflammation and support circulation.

TURMERIC AND BLACK PEPPER TEA

Boosts anti-inflammatory response.

Ingredients

- 1 tsp turmeric powder
- Pinch of black pepper
- 1 cup hot water

Instructions

- Mix ingredients and allow to steep for 10 minutes. Drink once daily.

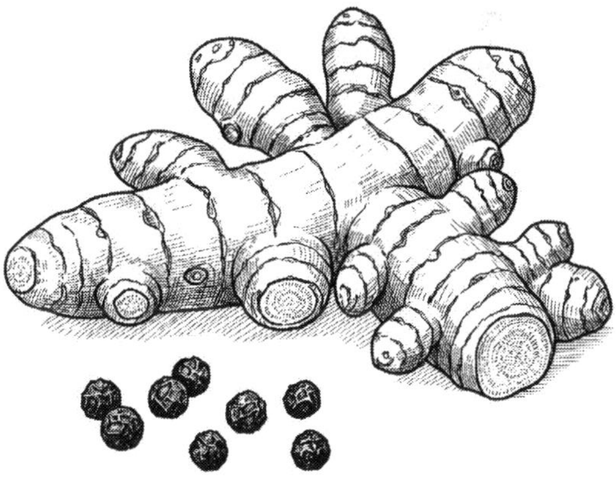

NETTLE LEAF AND LEMON BALM TEA

Helps reduce inflammation while calming the nervous system.

Ingredients

- 1 tsp dried nettle leaf
- 1 tsp dried lemon balm
- 1 cup hot water

Instructions

- Steep the nettle and lemon balm in hot water for 10 minutes. Strain and sip slowly.

GENERAL PAIN RELIEF: HERBAL POULTICES FOR LOCALIZED PAIN

Whether it's from an injury, stress, or chronic conditions, pain can take a serious toll on your well-being. But the good news is that poultices can offer effective relief, helping to soothe the pain, reduce inflammation, and promote healing.

GINGER POULTICE

Stimulates circulation and relieves pain.

Ingredients

- 2 tbsp grated ginger
- 1 cloth

Instructions

- Wrap ginger in a cloth and apply to painful areas. Do not use for extended periods (longer than a week) as it may lead to bruises forming easily.

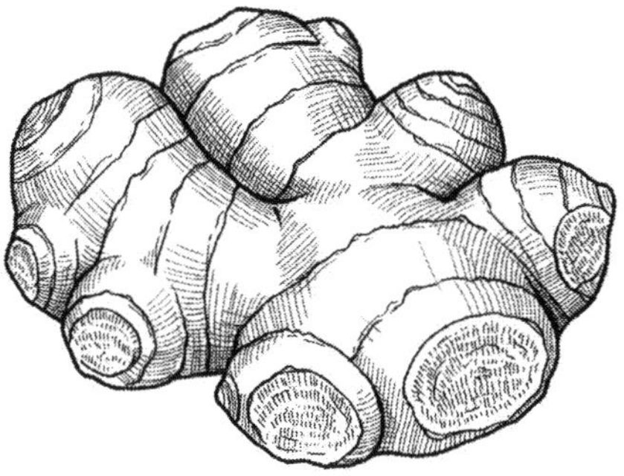

COMFREY POULTICE

Promotes healing and reduces pain and swelling.

Ingredients

- 2 tbsp dried comfrey leaves
- Warm water
- 1 gauze or cheesecloth

Instructions

- Add warm water to the comfrey leaves to create a thick paste. Apply the paste to a gauze or cheesecloth. Allow the poultice to sit on the painful area for half an hour. Repeat up to three times a day for relief.

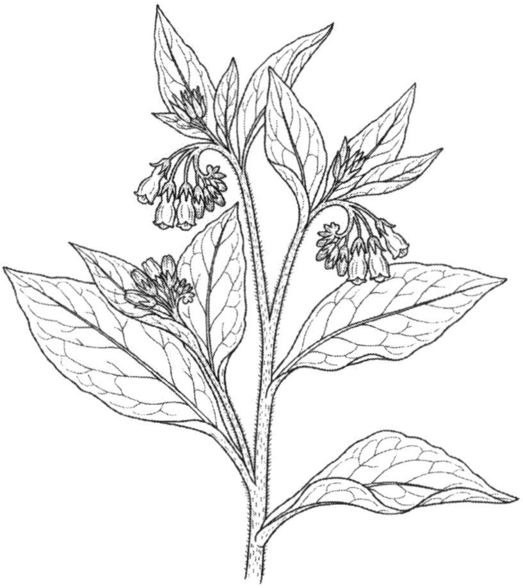

CHAPTER 10:

SLEEP AND STRESS REMEDIES

Sleep and stress are deeply connected – lack of sleep can heighten stress, while stress can make it harder to fall asleep. Herbal and natural remedies can help by promoting relaxation, easing anxiety, and supporting restful sleep.

INSOMNIA: HERBAL TEAS FOR SLEEP INDUCTION

Certain herbal teas can help induce sleep by calming the nervous system.

CHAMOMILE TEA

Promotes relaxation and supports deep sleep.

For detailed brewing instructions, see Chapter Seven, *Gas and Bloating: Carminative Herbal Remedies.*

VALERIAN ROOT TEA

Reduces the time it takes to fall asleep.

Ingredients

- 1 tsp dried valerian root
- 1 cup hot water

Instructions

- Steep the ingredients for 10 minutes while covered. Strain and drink roughly half an hour before sleeping.

PASSIONFLOWER TEA

Promotes calmness and reduces nighttime anxiety.

Ingredients

- 1 tsp dried passionflower
- 1 cup hot water

Instructions

- Steep passionflower for 10 minutes while covered. Strain and drink before bed.

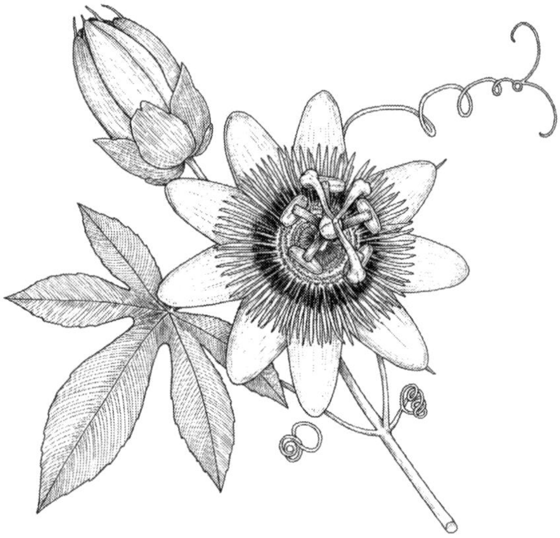

CALIFORNIA POPPY TEA

Encourages relaxation and supports deeper sleep cycles.

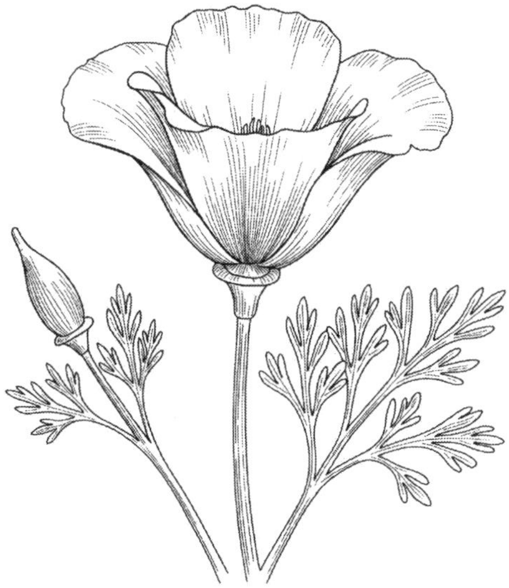

Ingredients

- 1 tsp dried California poppy
- 1 cup hot water

Instructions

- Steep for 10–15 minutes. Strain and sweeten with honey if desired. Drink the tea 30 minutes before bed. Do not drink more than one cup a day, and do not use the remedy if you need to drive or perform a task that needs your full attention.

HOPS AND LEMON BALM TEA

Eases restlessness and promotes deep, uninterrupted sleep.

Ingredients

- 1 tsp dried hops flowers
- 1 tsp dried lemon balm
- 1 cup hot water

Instructions

- Steep the ingredients in hot water for 10 minutes. Don't forget to keep it covered while steeping. Strain and drink the tea 30 minutes before bed.

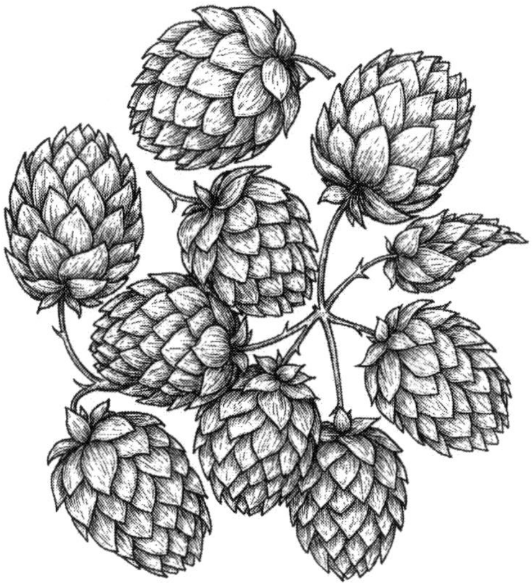

ASHWAGANDHA AND NUTMEG SLEEP TONIC

Helps the body unwind, promoting restful sleep.

Ingredients

- 1 tsp dried ashwagandha root
- Pinch of freshly grated nutmeg
- 1 cup hot milk (dairy or plant-based)

Instructions

- Simmer ashwagandha in milk for five minutes. Remove from heat, add nutmeg, and drink warm half an hour before bed.

MAGNESIUM AND OAT STRAW SLEEP-ENHANCING TEA

Supports muscle relaxation and deep sleep.

Ingredients

- 1 tsp oat straw
- 1 tsp chamomile
- 1 tsp lemon balm
- 1 cup hot water
- ¼ tsp magnesium citrate powder (stir in after steeping)

Instructions

- Steep the ingredients for 10 minutes in hot water. Strain, add magnesium, and drink before bed.

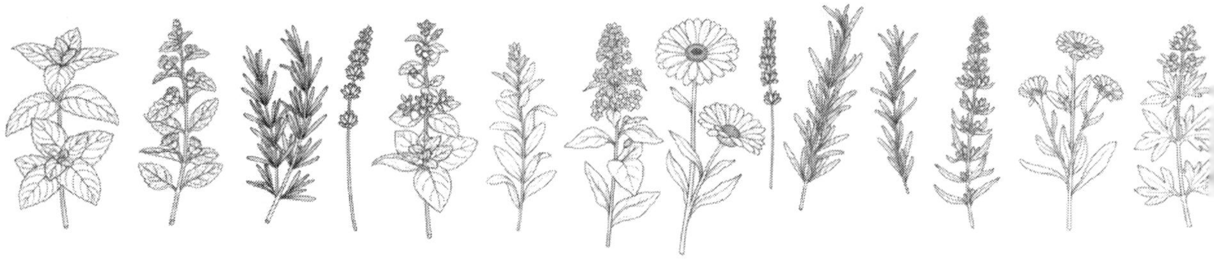

ANXIETY: HERBAL REMEDIES FOR CALMING THE MIND

These remedies can help reduce stress and support mental clarity with consistent use.

LEMON BALM TEA

Eases nervous restlessness and improves mood.

Ingredients

- 1 tsp dried or fresh lemon balm leaves
- 1 cup of hot water

Instructions

- Place the lemon balm in a cup and pour hot water over. Cover the cup and allow the herb to infuse for 10 minutes. Strain and sweeten with honey if desired. For best results, enjoy a cup of lemon balm at night, as it has mild sedative properties.

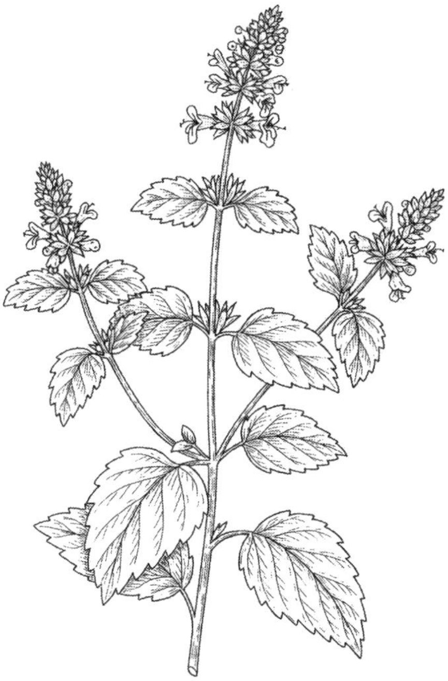

ASHWAGANDHA TINCTURE

Supports stress resilience and reduces stress levels.

Ingredients

- 1 cup dried ashwagandha root (cut or powdered)
- 2 cups high-proof alcohol (vodka or brandy, at least 80 proof)

Instructions

- Add the ashwagandha root to a clean glass and top with alcohol. The herb must be fully submerged. Close the jar tightly and store it in a cool, dark place for six weeks. When the tincture is ready, strain and transfer the liquid into a dark glass dropper bottle. Store it in a cool, dark place. To use, take 30 drops in water once a day. This tincture is best used at night.

ROSE PETAL AND OAT STRAW TEA

Calms frazzled nerves and nourishes the nervous system.

Ingredients

- 1 tbsp dried rose petals
- 1 tbsp oat straw
- 1 cup hot water

Instructions

- Combine rose petals and oat straw in a cup. Pour hot water over and steep for 15 minutes while covered. Drink once daily to support emotional well-being.

LAVENDER ESSENTIAL OIL

Reduces nervous tension and promotes calmness.

Ingredients

- 5-10 drops of lavender essential oil

Instructions

- To apply lavender essential oil to the pulse points, dilute five drops in a tablespoon of carrier oil (jojoba, avocado, or grapeseed works well), then massage into the temples, wrists, and behind the ears. Use as often as needed.
- Drop two to three drops of lavender essential oil onto your pillow case before sleeping to encourage restful sleep.
- Alternatively, place 5-10 drops of the essential oil into a diffuser and allow the calming aroma to permeate your bedroom.

HOLY BASIL (TULSI) TINCTURE

Promotes relaxation and balances stress hormones.

Ingredients

- 1 cup fresh or ½ cup dried holy basil leaves
- 2 cups high-proof alcohol (vodka or brandy, at least 80 proof)

Instructions

- Place the holy basil in a jar. Pour in the alcohol, making sure the leaves are fully submerged. Store the sealed jar in a cupboard or any other cool, dark place for six weeks. Afterwards, strain the tincture and transfer it into a dropper bottle. To use, take 30 drops in water up to twice daily to ease stress and promote calmness.

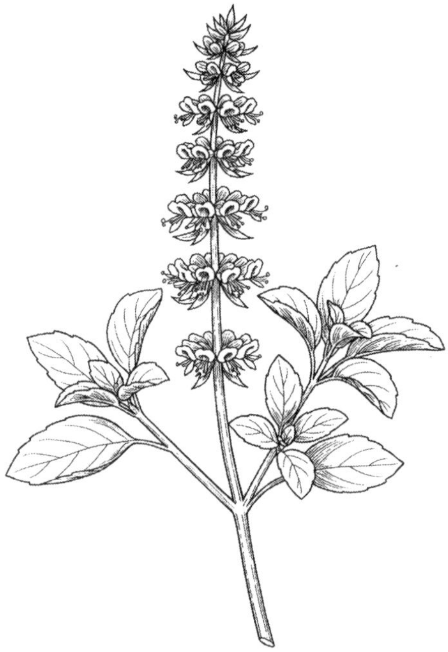

BLUE VERVAIN TINCTURE

Eases nervous tension, soothes frazzled nerves, and supports emotional balance.

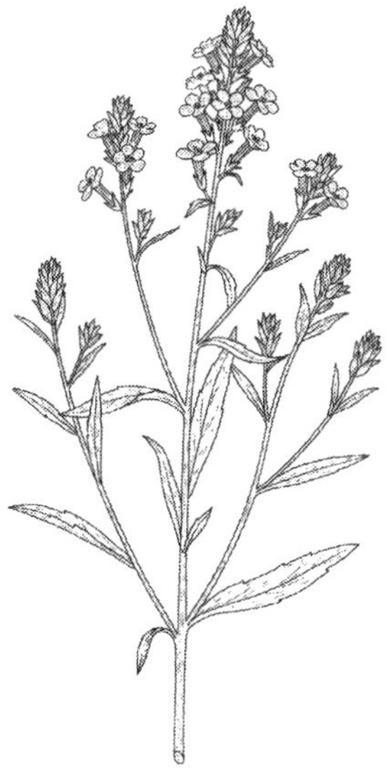

Ingredients

- 1 cup fresh blue vervain leaves and flowers (or ½ cup dried)
- 2 cups high-proof alcohol (vodka or brandy, at least 80 proof)

Instructions

- Place the blue vervain in a clean glass jar. Fill with alcohol, ensuring the plant material is fully submerged. For six weeks, you'll need to keep the jar in a cool, dark place to infuse. Strain the tincture through a fine strainer or cheesecloth, squeezing out excess liquid. Transfer to a dark glass dropper. Take 20–30 drops in water up to twice daily for stress relief and relaxation.

AROMATHERAPY FOR ANXIETY RELIEF

Using essential oils through inhalation can quickly calm the nervous system and ease anxiety.

Ingredients

- 4 drops lavender essential oil
- 3 drops bergamot essential oil
- 2 drops frankincense essential oil
- Bowl of steaming water or an essential oil diffuser

Instructions

- Add the essential oils to a bowl of steaming water. Drape a towel over your head to trap as much steam as possible and inhale for 5–10 minutes. Alternatively, you can add the essential oils to a diffuser and allow the calming aroma to fill the room.
- For anxiety relief on the go, simply add the oils to a small inhaler and breathe in as needed. Alternatively, blend the essential oils with a tablespoon of carrier oil (such as jojoba or avocado) and pour into a small roll-on applicator bottle. Apply to your pulse points as needed.

STRESS-INDUCED INSOMNIA: HERBAL BLENDS FOR DUAL RELIEF

These blends help ease stress while promoting restful sleep. *For optimal results, pair these remedies with calming activities, like deep breathing or meditation.*

CHAMOMILE AND LAVENDER TEA

Calms the nervous system and supports deep sleep.

Ingredients

- 1 tsp dried chamomile flowers
- ½ tsp dried lavender flowers
- 1 cup hot water

Instructions

- Combine chamomile and lavender in a tea infuser or teapot. Pour hot water over the herbs and steep for 10–15 minutes, covered. Drink the tea before bed. Do not drink more than one cup a day.

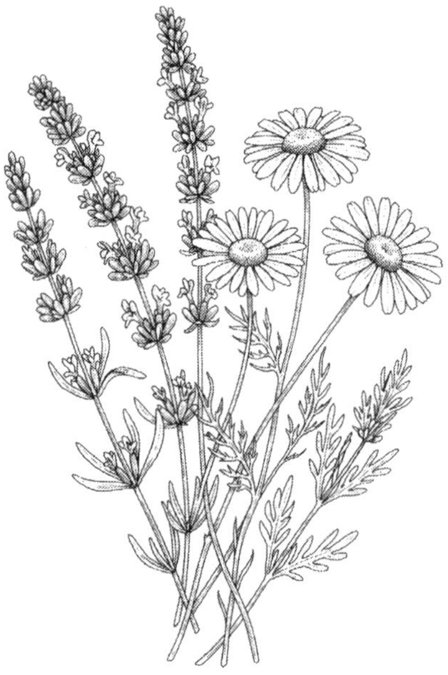

VALERIAN AND HOPS TEA

Enhances relaxation and shortens sleep onset time.

Ingredients

- 1 tsp dried valerian root
- ½ tsp dried hops flowers
- 1 cup hot water

Instructions

- Add valerian and hops to a teapot. Steep for 10 minutes. Strain and drink before bedtime.

PASSIONFLOWER AND LEMON BALM TEA

Reduces anxiety and helps maintain a steady sleep cycle.

Ingredients

- 1 tsp dried passionflower
- 1 tsp dried lemon balm
- 1 cup hot water

Instructions

- Place passionflower and lemon balm in a cup. Allow the herbs to steep for 10 minutes, then strain and sweeten with honey if needed. Drink the tea an hour before bed. Do not drink more than one cup per day.

CALIFORNIA POPPY AND SKULLCAP TINCTURE

Helps quiet a restless mind and ease stress-related insomnia.

Ingredients

- 1 cup dried California poppy
- 1 cup dried skullcap
- high-proof alcohol (vodka or brandy, at least 80 proof)

Instructions

- Fill a glass jar halfway with the dried herbs. Cover completely with alcohol, ensuring herbs are submerged. Store the jar for six weeks in a dark and cool place. Strain the liquid and store in a dark dropper bottle. Take 30 drops in water half an hour before bed.

HOLY BASIL AND ROSE TEA

Helps to soothe stress and reduce emotional tension.

Ingredients

- 1 tsp dried holy basil (tulsi)
- ½ tsp dried rose petals
- 1 cup hot water

Instructions

- Add holy basil and rose petals to a teapot or cup. Let the herbs steep for 10–15 minutes in hot water. Strain and sweeten with honey if desired. Drink the tea in the evening to unwind.

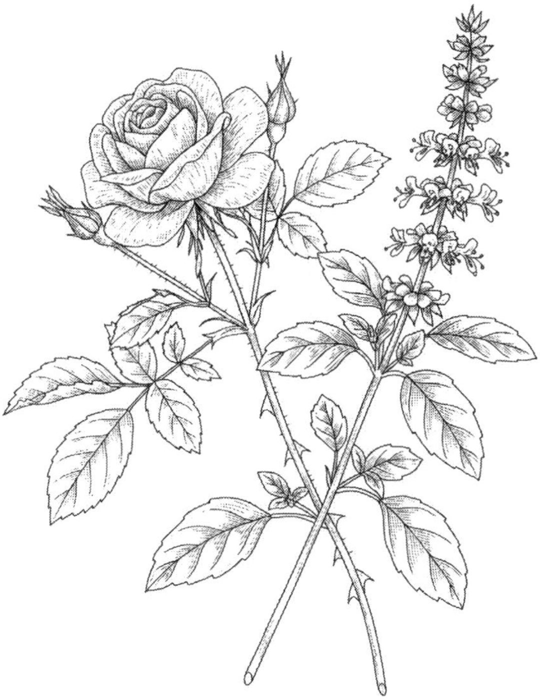

MORINGA AND CHAMOMILE NIGHTTIME TEA

Supports relaxation, reduces stress, and provides essential nutrients for restful sleep.

Ingredients

- 1 tsp dried moringa leaves
- 1 tsp dried chamomile flowers
- 1 cup hot water
- ½ tsp honey (optional)

Instructions

- Add moringa and chamomile to a teapot. Let the herbs steep for 10 minutes in hot water. Drink in the evening to promote relaxation and sleep.

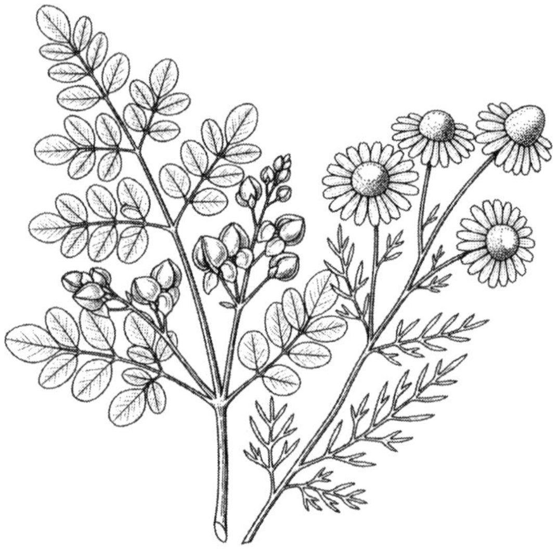

ASHWAGANDHA AND HOLY BASIL TEA

This calming tea blend can help to reduce stress, enhance mood, and promote a restful night's sleep.

Ingredients

- 1 tsp dried Ashwagandha root (or 1/2 tsp Ashwagandha powder)
- 1 tsp dried Holy Basil (Tulsi) leaves
- 1 cup hot water
- honey (optional, to taste)

Instructions

- Place the Ashwagandha root and Holy Basil leaves into a tea infuser or directly into your cup. Pour hot water (just below boiling) over the herbs. Cover and steep for 10–12 minutes to fully extract the beneficial compounds. Drink this tea 30–60 minutes before bed or when you're feeling stressed.

RESTLESS LEG SYNDROME: HERBAL REMEDIES FOR CALMING SENSATIONS

Certain herbs relax muscles and calm the nervous system to reduce leg discomfort.

PEPPERMINT TEA

Relaxes leg muscles and reduces tension.

For detailed brewing instructions, see Chapter Six, *Cold and Flu: Herbal Teas for Symptom Relief.*

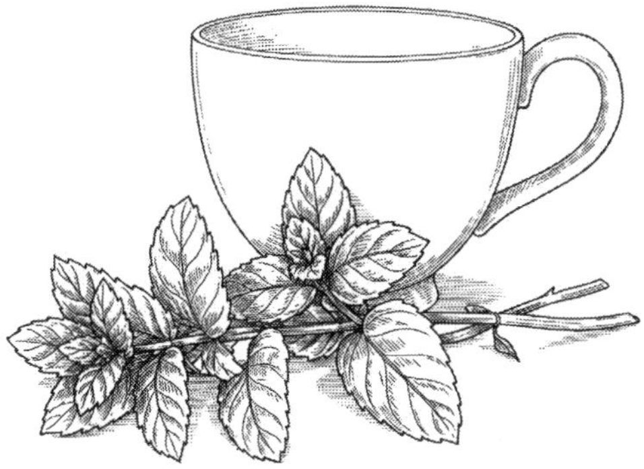

GINGER COMPRESS

Improves circulation and relieves muscle discomfort.

For detailed instructions, see Chapter Nine, *General Pain Relief: Herbal Poultices for Localized Pain.*

LAVENDER MASSAGE OIL

Soothes nighttime restlessness.

Ingredients

- 5-10 drops of lavender essential oil
- 1 tbsp of carrier oil (rosehip, avocado, or jojoba works well)

Instructions

- Dilute lavender essential oil in a carrier oil. Massage into legs before sleep.

EPSOM SALT SOAK

Relieves muscle spasms and calms the nervous system.

Ingredients

- 2 cups of Epsom salts

Instructions

- Add Epsom salts (magnesium sulfate) to warm bathwater. Soak for 20–30 minutes before bed to relax muscles and ease restless legs.

EPSOM SALT AND LAVENDER FOOT SOAK

Relieves muscle tension and promotes relaxation.

Ingredients

- 1 cup Epsom salt
- 5 drops of lavender essential oil
- Warm water

Instructions

- Fill a basin with warm water and add the Epsom salt and essential oil. Soak your feet for 20 minutes before bed to help relax your muscles and reduce discomfort in your legs.

VALERIAN ROOT AND CLOVE INFUSED OIL

Soothes muscle tension and relaxes the nervous system.

Ingredients

- 2 tbsp dried valerian root
- 1 tbsp ground cloves
- Half a cup olive oil (or carrier oil of choice)

Instructions

- In a double boiler, gently heat the olive oil and add the valerian root and ground clove. Allow the herbs to infuse into the oil for about 30 minutes, making sure the oil doesn't overheat. Once cooled, strain the oil and store it in a dark glass bottle. Massage the infused oil into your legs before bed to help calm restless muscles and reduce discomfort.

FENNEL AND LEMON BALM TEA

Helps soothe muscles and calm the nerves.

Ingredients

- 1 tsp fennel seeds
- 1 tsp dried lemon balm
- 1 cup hot water

Instructions

- Steep fennel and lemon balm in hot water for 10 minutes. Strain and drink before bed. Fennel helps with muscle relaxation, and lemon balm promotes calmness.

EPSOM SALT AND ROSEMARY FOOT SOAK

Helps relax muscles and ease tension in the legs and feet.

Ingredients

- 1 cup Epsom salt
- 5 drops rosemary essential oil
- Warm water (enough to cover your feet or legs)

Instructions

- Add warm water and Epsom salt to a basin. Stir until dissolved. Add the rosemary essential oil and stir again. Soak your feet or legs for 20–30 minutes before bed. The magnesium in Epsom salt helps relax muscles, while rosemary oil improves circulation and provides a soothing effect.

NIGHTMARES: HERBAL REMEDIES FOR PEACEFUL SLEEP

Herbal remedies can help prevent nightmares and encourage deep, uninterrupted sleep.

MUGWORT TEA

Promotes lucid dreaming and reduces nightmares.

Ingredients

- 1 tsp dried mugwort
- 1 cup hot water

Instructions

Steep mugwort in hot water for 10–15 minutes. Strain and drink 30 minutes before bed. It's best to start with a small amount to see how it affects your dreams.

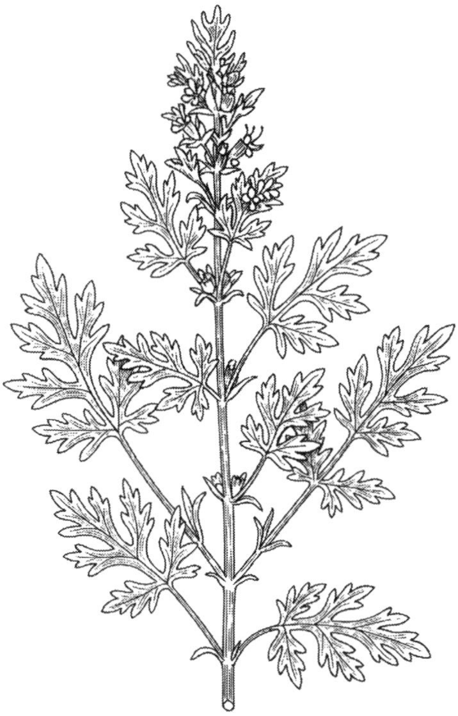

CHAMOMILE AND VALERIAN TEA

Eases subconscious anxiety contributing to bad dreams.

Ingredients

- 1 tsp dried chamomile flowers
- ½ tsp dried valerian root
- 1 cup hot water

Instructions

- Steep the chamomile and valerian root in hot water for 10–15 minutes. Strain and drink an hour before bed. Valerian has a strong taste – add honey if needed.

HOLY BASIL AND LICORICE ROOT TEA

Reduces stress and fear-based nightmares.

Ingredients

- 1 tsp dried holy basil
- ½ tsp dried licorice root
- 1 cup hot water

Instructions

- Steep herbs in hot water for 10–15 minutes. Strain and drink 30 minutes before bed. Do not drink more than one cup a day.

CEDARWOOD AND SANDALWOOD DIFFUSION MIX

Grounding essential oils to prevent unsettling dreams.

Ingredients

- 4 drops cedarwood essential oil
- 3 drops sandalwood essential oil
- diffuser

Instructions

- Add essential oils to a diffuser filled with water. Run the diffuser for 30 minutes before bed. These earthy scents promote a sense of safety and relaxation.

BANANA AND NUTMEG SLEEP SMOOTHIE

Promotes deep sleep and relaxation.

Ingredients

- 1 ripe banana
- 1 cup warm almond milk (or milk of choice)
- ¼ tsp ground nutmeg
- 1 tsp honey (optional)

Instructions

- Blend all ingredients until smooth. Drink 30–60 minutes before bed. Nutmeg has mild sedative properties, and banana provides natural sleep-supporting magnesium.

LAVENDER SACHET

Enhances relaxation when placed under your pillow.

Ingredients

- 2 tbsp dried lavender flowers
- small fabric sachet or muslin bag

Instructions

- Fill a sachet with dried lavender flowers. Place it under your pillow or near your bedside. Refresh every few weeks for maximum effect.

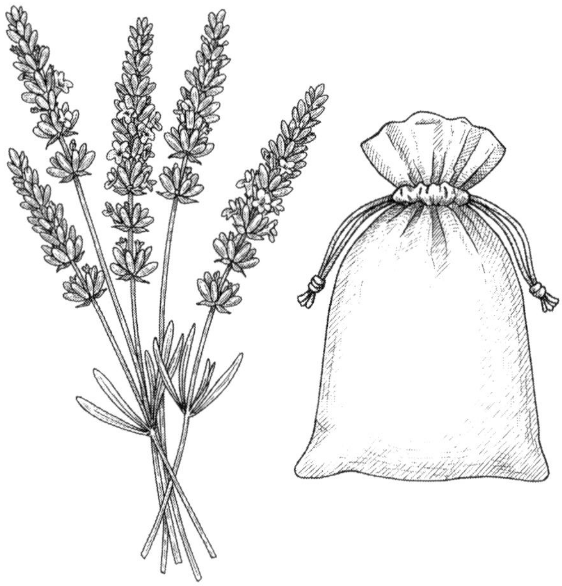

ROSE AND CHAMOMILE PILLOW MIST

Promotes emotional balance and peaceful sleep.

Ingredients

- ½ cup distilled water
- 1 tbsp witch hazel
- 5 drops chamomile essential oil
- 3 drops rose essential oil
- small spray bottle

Instructions

- Mix all ingredients in a spray bottle. Lightly mist over your pillow before bedtime. Shake well before each use.

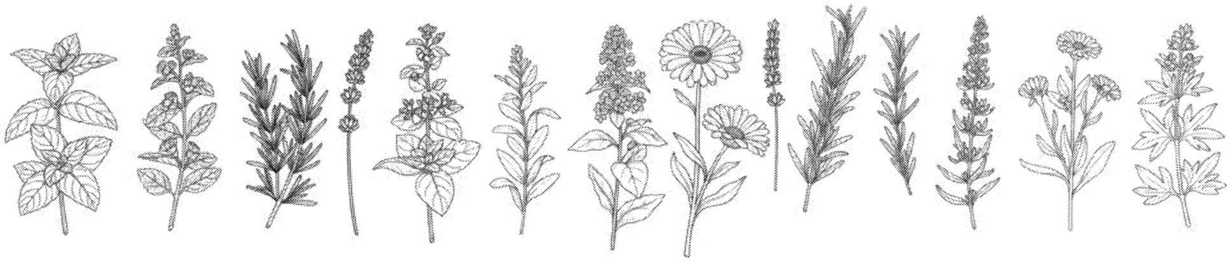

STRESS-RELATED DIGESTIVE ISSUES: HERBAL TEAS FOR SOOTHING THE GUT

Stress can disrupt digestion; these herbs help relax the digestive tract and reduce bloating, nausea, and discomfort.

PEPPERMINT TEA

Soothes stress-induced bloating and irritable bowel symptoms.

For detailed brewing instructions, see Chapter Six, *Cold and Flu: Herbal Teas for Symptom Relief.*

GINGER TEA

Relieves stress-related nausea and aids digestion.

For detailed brewing instructions, see Chapter Six, *Cold and Flu: Herbal Teas for Symptom Relief.*

CHAMOMILE TEA

Relaxes the gut and soothes nervous stomach discomfort.

For detailed brewing instructions, see Chapter Seven, *Gas and Bloating: Carminative Herbal Remedies.*

MARSHMALLOW ROOT AND LICORICE TEA

Coats the stomach lining, reducing acid reflux and stress-induced irritation.

Ingredients

- 1 tsp dried marshmallow root
- ½ tsp dried licorice root
- 1 cup warm (not boiling) water

Instructions:

- Steep herbs in warm water for 15 minutes. Strain and sip slowly before or after meals. Avoid licorice if you have high blood pressure.

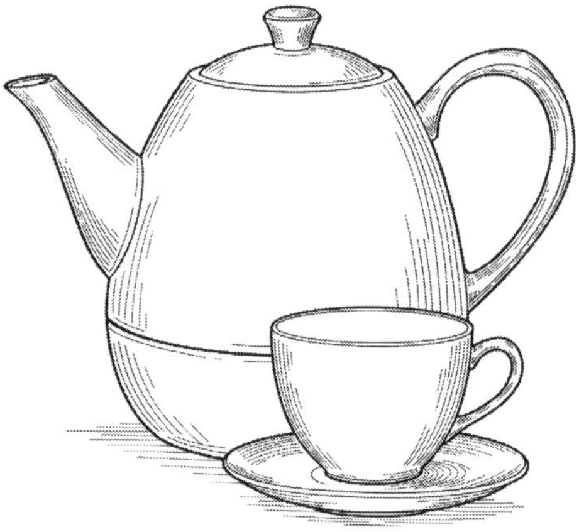

CARDAMOM AND ROSE TEA

Relaxes the digestive tract and uplifts the mood while easing stress-induced indigestion.

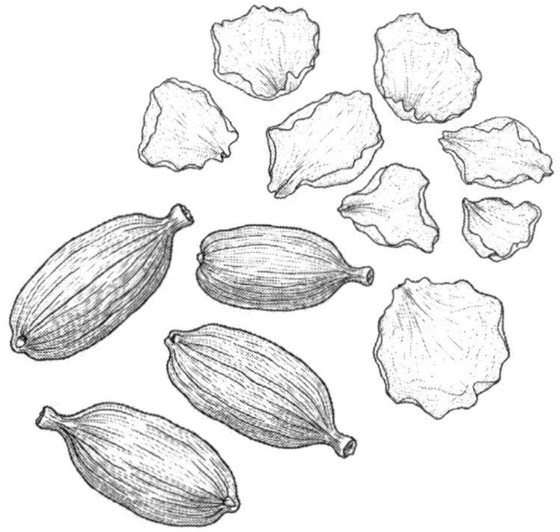

Ingredients

- 3 crushed cardamom pods
- 1 tsp dried rose petals
- 1 cup hot water

Instructions

- Steep herbs in hot water for 10 minutes. Strain and drink between meals to ease discomfort.

SLIPPERY ELM AND CHAMOMILE TEA

Coats the stomach lining, reducing irritation and stress-induced digestive upset.

Ingredients

- 1 tsp slippery elm powder
- 1 tsp dried chamomile
- 1 cup warm (not boiling) water

Instructions

- Mix slippery elm powder with warm water and let sit for a few minutes. Steep chamomile separately in warm water for 10 minutes, then strain. Combine the two teas and drinks before bed or after meals for a soothing effect.

CATNIP AND GINGER TEA

Relaxes digestive spasms, soothes nausea, and reduces stress-related gut discomfort.

Ingredients

- 1 tsp dried catnip leaves
- ½ tsp grated fresh ginger
- 1 cup hot water

Instructions

- Steep catnip and ginger in hot water for 10 minutes. Strain and drink before or after meals to ease digestion and calm the nerves. Ginger has a strong taste, so sweeten the tea with honey if needed.

TENSION HEADACHES: HERBAL REMEDIES FOR RELIEF

Tension headaches are the most common type of headache, often caused by stress, anxiety, poor posture, or muscle tension. These herbal remedies can help relieve headaches caused by stress and anxiety.

PEPPERMINT MASSAGE OIL

Relieves muscle tension and headache pain.

Ingredients

- 2 drops peppermint essential oil
- 1 teaspoon carrier oil (coconut, almond, or jojoba oil)

Instructions

- Dilute peppermint essential oil in a carrier oil and apply it to your temples, the back of your neck, and behind your ears. Gently massage these areas in circular motions for a few minutes to ease tension. Inhale the refreshing aroma deeply to enhance relaxation.
- For an extra soothing effect, rub a drop or two of the diluted oil between your palms, cup your hands over your nose, and inhale deeply for three to five minutes.
- For on-the-go relief, store the diluted oil in a small roll-on bottle and apply as needed. Do not use this remedy for young children.

FEVERFEW TEA

Prevents and reduces headache severity.

Ingredients

- 1 teaspoon dried feverfew leaves (or three fresh leaves)
- 1 cup hot water
- honey (optional)

Instructions

- Steep feverfew leaves in hot water for 10 minutes. Strain and drink once daily to help prevent headaches. Sweeten with honey if desired.

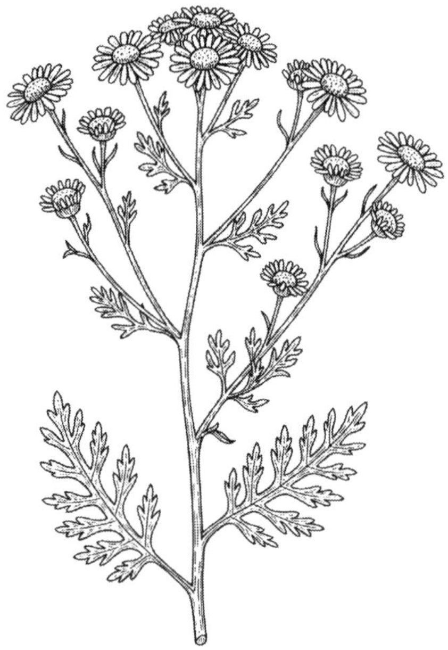

GINGER TEA

Reduces inflammation and headache triggers.

For detailed brewing instructions, see Chapter Six, *Cold and Flu: Herbal Teas for Symptom Relief.*

EUCALYPTUS AND LEMON BALM AROMATHERAPY

Clears the mind, reduces stress, and eases tension.

Ingredients

- 3 drops eucalyptus essential oil
- 3 drops lemon balm (Melissa) essential oil
- Bowl of hot water (or diffuser)

Instructions

- Add eucalyptus and lemon balm essential oils to a bowl of hot water or a diffuser. Inhale the steam deeply for 5-10 minutes to promote relaxation and relieve headache discomfort. For an extra calming effect, apply diluted lemon balm oil to your temples.

ROSEMARY AND PEPPERMINT STEAM INHALATION

Relaxes muscles and relieves headache pain.

Ingredients

- 1 tablespoon dried rosemary leaves (or two fresh sprigs)
- 1 tablespoon dried peppermint leaves (or five fresh leaves)
- 4 cups boiling water

Instructions

- Pour boiling water over rosemary and peppermint leaves in a bowl. Loosely drape a towel over your head and shoulders and use it as a makeshift "tent" to wrap the steam. Inhale deeply for 10 minutes. Repeat as often as needed.

MAGNESIUM-RICH HERBAL INFUSION

Eases muscle tension and supports relaxation.

Ingredients

- 1 teaspoon dried nettle leaves
- 1 teaspoon dried oat straw
- 1 cup hot water

Instructions

- Steep nettle and oat straw in hot water for 10 minutes. Strain and drink once a day to relieve muscle tension and headaches naturally.

ADRENAL FATIGUE: HERBAL REMEDIES FOR ENERGY RESTORATION

These herbs help to restore energy and balance stress hormones to prevent burnout.

LICORICE ROOT TEA

Helps maintain healthy adrenal function and promotes balanced cortisol levels.

Ingredients

- 1 teaspoon dried licorice root
- 1 cup hot water
- honey (optional)

Instructions

Steep licorice root in hot water for 10 minutes. Strain and drink in the morning. Sweeten with honey if desired. Avoid prolonged use if you have high blood pressure.

RHODIOLA ROSEA TEA

Enhances mental and physical endurance during stress.

Ingredients

- 1 teaspoon dried rhodiola root
- 1 cup hot water
- lemon or honey (optional)

Instructions

- Steep rhodiola root in hot water for 10-15 minutes. Strain and drink in the morning or early afternoon for an energy boost. Add lemon or honey if desired.

ASHWAGANDHA INFUSION

Improves stress resilience and balances energy levels.

Ingredients

- 1 teaspoon dried ashwagandha root (or ½ teaspoon ashwagandha powder)
- 1 cup hot water
- honey or cinnamon (optional)

Instructions

- Steep ashwagandha in hot water for 10-15 minutes. Strain and drink in the evening to support relaxation and energy balance. Add honey or cinnamon if desired.

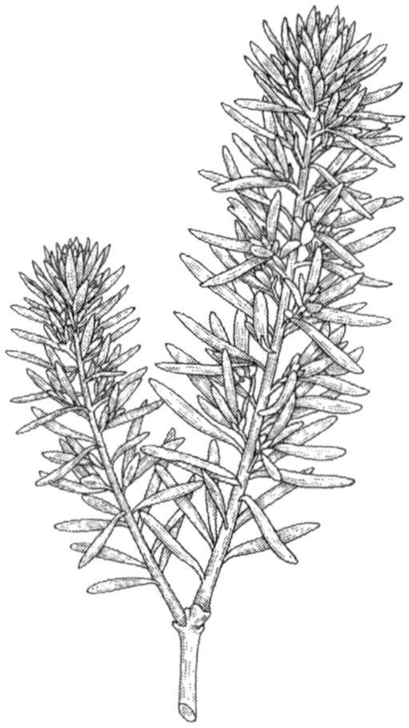

SCHISANDRA BERRY TONIC

Supports adrenal function and increases resistance to stress.

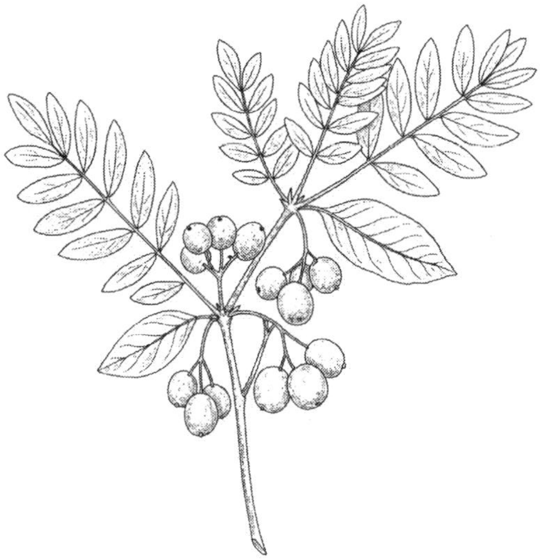

Ingredients

- 1 teaspoon dried schisandra berries
- 1 cup hot water
- honey (optional)

Instructions

- Simmer schisandra berries in hot water for 10 minutes. Strain and drink once daily to improve energy and mental clarity.

MACA ROOT SMOOTHIE

Balances hormones and increases sustained energy.

Ingredients

- 1 teaspoon maca root powder
- 1 cup almond or oat milk½ banana
- 1 teaspoon honey
- ¼ teaspoon cinnamon

Instructions

- Blend all ingredients until smooth. Drink in the morning to naturally boost energy and support adrenal function.

NETTLE LEAF INFUSION

Nourishes the adrenal glands and replenishes essential minerals.

Ingredients

- 1 tablespoon dried nettle leaves
- 2 cups hot water

Instructions

- Steep nettle leaves in hot water for 15-20 minutes. Strain and drink throughout the day to restore energy and support adrenal function.

PANIC ATTACKS: HERBAL REMEDIES FOR IMMEDIATE CALM

Calming natural remedies can help reduce the intensity of panic attacks and restore emotional harmony.

LAVENDER ESSENTIAL OIL

Can help calm the nervous system.

For detailed usage suggestions, see *Anxiety: Herbal Remedies for Calming the Mind*. For best results, pair with a lavender sachet under the pillow and lavender massage oil for lasting relief.

SKULLCAP TINCTURE

Reduces nervous excitability.

For detailed instructions on how to create the tincture, see Chapter Nine, *Nerve Pain: Herbal Remedies for Neuropathic Relief.*

LEMON BALM TEA

Stops racing thoughts and eases panic symptoms.

Ingredients

- 1 to 2 teaspoons dried lemon balm leaves (or 3-4 fresh leaves)
- 1 cup hot water
- honey or lemon (optional)

Instructions

- Add the dried or fresh lemon balm leaves to a cup. Steep the leaves in hot water for 5-10 minutes. Strain the tea and sweeten with honey or add a slice of lemon if desired. Drink once or twice daily to help ease stress and promote relaxation.

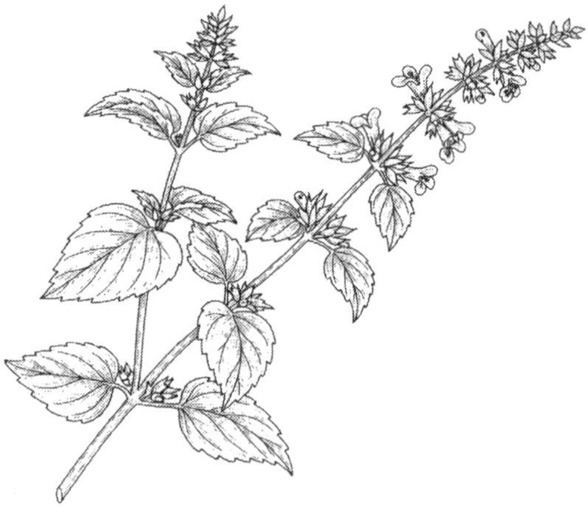

EMOTIONAL STRESS AND OVERWHELM: HERBAL SUPPORT FOR NERVOUS SYSTEM RESILIENCE

Some herbs support and strengthen the nervous system, helping you better adapt to stress and build resilience over time.

HOLY BASIL TEA

Reduces mental fatigue and regulates stress hormones.

For detailed brewing instructions, see Chapter Seven, *Gas and Bloating: Carminative Herbal Remedies.*

OAT STRAW INFUSION

Nourishes the nervous system for long-term stress support.

Ingredients

- 1 tablespoon dried oat straw (Avena sativa)
- 1 cup boiling water

Instructions

- Place the oat straw in a heatproof jar or teapot. Pour boiling water over and let it steep covered for 15-20 minutes. Strain the infusion to remove the oat straw leaves. Drink up to two cups daily, especially during times of stress, to help support the nervous system and promote long-term resilience.

ROSE PETAL TEA

Promotes emotional balance and heart-centered relaxation.

Ingredients

- 1-2 teaspoons dried rose petals (organic, preferably fragrant)
- 1 cup hot water
- honey or lemon (optional)

Instructions

- Add dried rose petals to a cup or teapot. Pour hot (not boiling) water over the petals. The water should be just below boiling to preserve the delicate flavor and nutrients. Cover the cup or teapot and let it steep for five minutes. Strain the tea and add honey or a slice of lemon for added flavor.

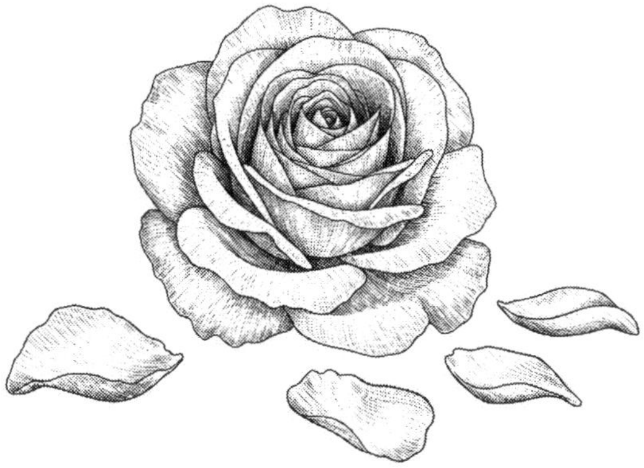

RED CLOVER BLOSSOM INFUSION

Gentle and restorative for emotional overwhelm and hormonal balance.

Ingredients

- 1 tablespoon dried red clover blossoms
- 1 cup hot water

Instructions

- Place dried red clover blossoms in a teapot and pour boiling water over the blossoms. Cover and steep for 10-15 minutes. Strain the tea and drink up to two cups daily for emotional support and to alleviate stress.

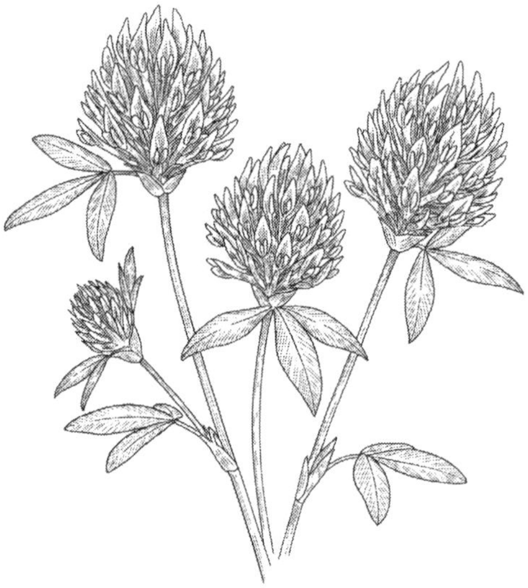

AROMATHERAPY WITH BERGAMOT AND YLANG YLANG

An uplifting aromatherapy blend to reduce emotional stress, promote calmness, and support emotional balance.

Ingredients

- 3 drops bergamot essential oil
- 3 drops ylang ylang essential oil
- a diffuser or a bowl of hot water

Instructions

- In a diffuser or bowl of hot water, add bergamot and ylang ylang essential oils. Let the aroma permeate the room for 15-20 minutes. Use this aromatherapy blend whenever you need emotional support, calm, and relaxation during stressful moments.

LAVENDER AND LEMON BALM OXYMEL

A powerful tonic that combines the healing properties of apple cider vinegar and herbal infusions to support emotional relaxation.

Ingredients

- 1 tablespoon dried lavender flowers
- 1 tablespoon dried lemon balm leaves
- 1/4 cup raw apple cider vinegar
- 1/4 cup honey (preferably raw or local)
- 1 cup water (for infusing herbs)

Instructions

- In a small saucepan, bring the water to a simmer. Add the herbs and allow the mixture to steep for 10-15 minutes, then strain the liquid into a jar. Stir apple cider vinegar and honey into the liquid. Stir well until the honey is dissolved. Take up to two tablespoons of the oxymel once or twice daily, or when feeling stressed and overwhelmed. You can dilute it with water or enjoy it as is. Store the oxymel in a sealed jar in the fridge.

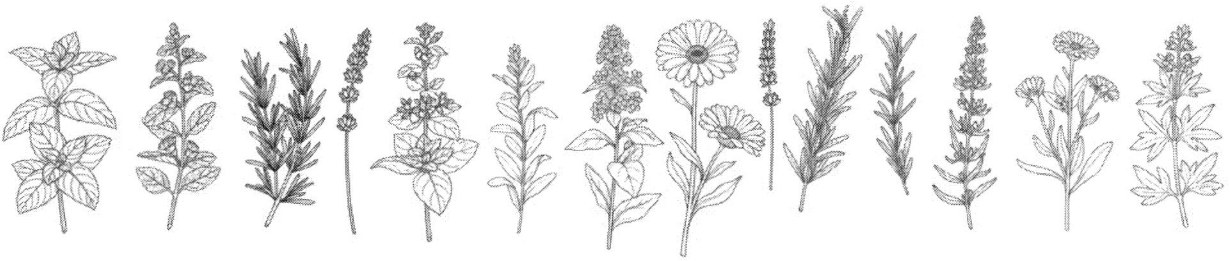

CHAPTER 11:

HORMONES AND WOMEN'S HEALTH

Hormones are the body's natural messengers, keeping everything from energy levels to mood, menstrual cycles, and menopause running smoothly. But when they fall out of sync, things can get a little frustrating – hello, PMS, irregular periods, fatigue, breakouts, and mood swings. The good news? There are natural remedies that can help restore balance, ease discomfort, and support overall reproductive health, because feeling good shouldn't be a struggle.

MENSTRUAL CYCLE SUPPORT: HERBAL TEAS FOR BALANCE

From easing cramps to calming PMS symptoms, these natural remedies support your body and keep things running smoothly.

RED RASPBERRY LEAF TEA

Traditionally used to tone the uterus, regulate cycles, and support fertility.

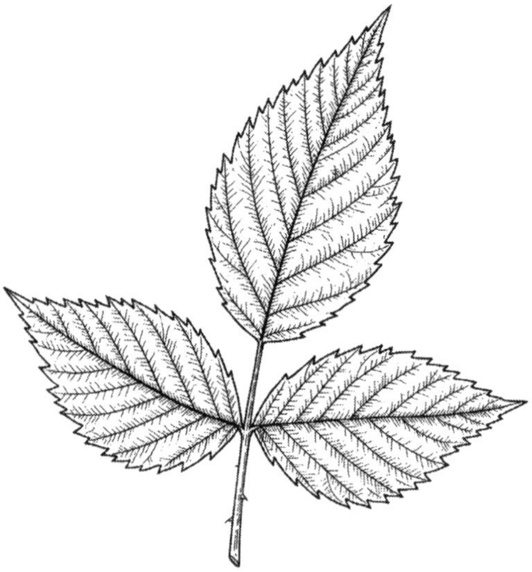

Ingredients

- 1 tsp dried red raspberry leaf
- 1 cup hot water

Instructions

- Place the leaves in a teapot and pour hot water over. Cover and steep for 10–15 minutes. Strain and drink once or twice daily.

SPEARMINT TEA

May help balance hormones, especially for women with high androgen levels.

Ingredients

- 1 tsp dried or fresh spearmint leaves
- 1 cup hot water

Instructions

- Place the herb in a teapot, pour hot water over and cover. Allow a steeping time of 5–10 minutes. Strain and drink twice daily. Avoid use if you are allergic to the mint family.

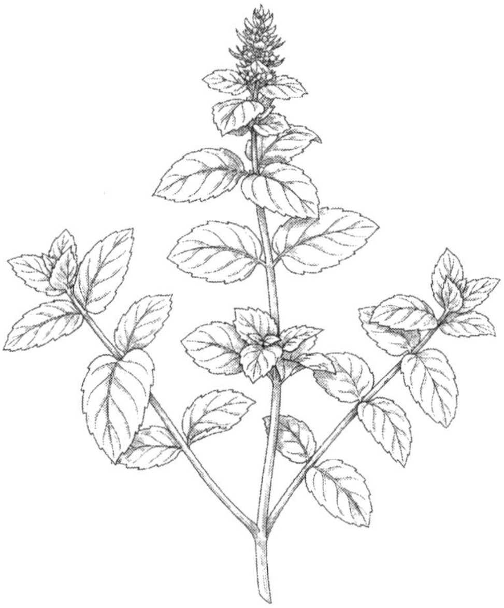

GINGER TEA

Supports circulation to the uterus and helps reduce painful cramps

For detailed brewing instructions, see Chapter Six, *Cold and Flu: Herbal Teas for Symptom Relief.*

DONG QUAI AND RASPBERRY LEAF TEA

Supports menstrual regularity and promotes circulation to reproductive organs.

Ingredients

- 1 tsp dried dong quai root
- 1 tsp dried red raspberry leaf
- 1 cup hot water

Instructions

- Place the herbs in a teapot and pour hot water over. Cover and steep for 15 minutes. Strain the tea and enjoy a cup twice a day during your period.

MUGWORT AND YARROW TEA

A traditional remedy for encouraging regular menstruation and easing stagnation in the uterus.

Ingredients

- 1 tsp dried mugwort
- 1 tsp dried yarrow
- 1 cup hot water

Instructions

- Place the herbs in a cup or teapot. Pour hot water over and steep covered for 10–15 minutes. Strain and drink once daily in the week, leading up to menstruation. Avoid this remedy during pregnancy, as these herbs can stimulate the uterus.

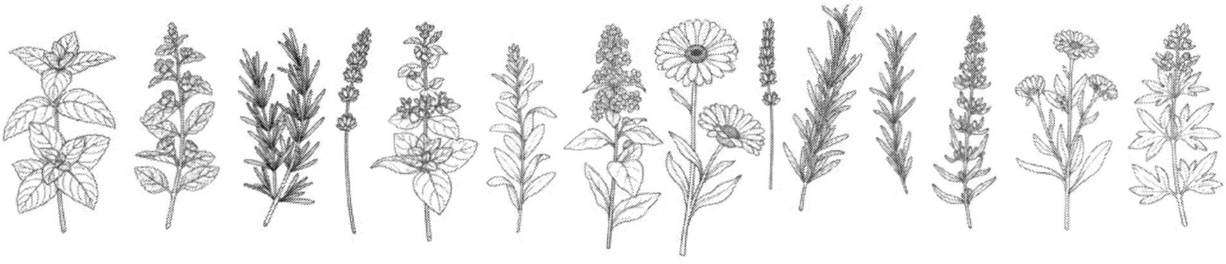

PMS AND MOOD SWINGS: HERBAL TINCTURES FOR HORMONAL HARMONY

These powerful tinctures can help to ease mood swings, hormonal tension, and feelings of irritability before menstruation.

PASSIONFLOWER TINCTURE

Relieves hormonal anxiety and promotes restful sleep.

Ingredients

- 1 cup dried passionflower
- 4 cups 80-proof alcohol (vodka or brandy)

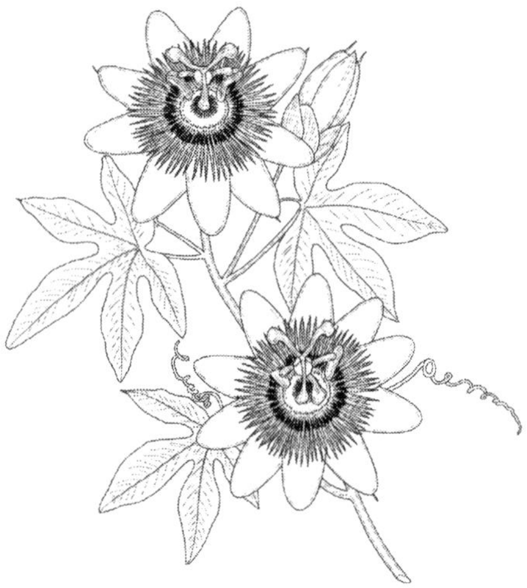

Instructions

- Fill a glass jar with dried passionflower. Submerge the herb with alcohol. Seal the jar tightly and store in a cool, dark place for six weeks. Strain when ready. To use, take 20 drops before bed.

LEMON BALM TINCTURE

Calms stress and supports emotional balance.

Ingredients

- 1 cup dried lemon balm leaves
- 4 cups 80-proof alcohol

Instructions

- Place dried lemon balm in a clean glass jar and pour alcohol over the herb, ensuring it's fully submerged. Seal the jar and shake it gently. Store in a cool, dark place for six weeks. Afterwards, strain the tincture into a clean container. Store in a dark glass dropper bottle for easy use. Take 20–30 drops up to three times daily.

CHASTEBERRY (VITEX) TINCTURE

Supports progesterone levels, reduces PMS symptoms, and promotes cycle regularity.

Ingredients

- 1 cup dried chasteberry (Vitex)
- 4 cups 80-proof alcohol (vodka or brandy works well)

Instructions

- Place dried chasteberry in a clean glass jar, filling it halfway. Cover the herbs with alcohol. Close the lid tightly and keep the jar tucked away in a cool, dark spot. Give it a good shake once a day for the next six weeks to help the infusion along. When it's ready, strain out the herbs and transfer the liquid to a dark glass dropper bottle. Take 30–40 drops in water each morning.

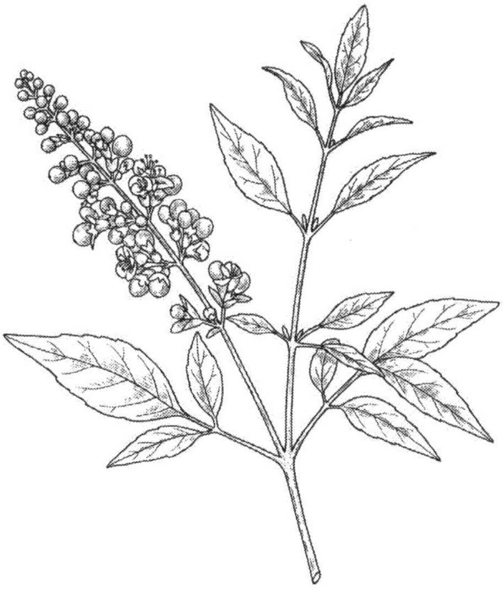

EVENING PRIMROSE OIL

May help regulate hormones, ease PMS symptoms, and support skin hydration.

Ingredients

- evening primrose oil supplements (usually comes in softgel capsules or liquid form)

Instructions:

- Follow the directions on the bottle, but do not exceed a dosage of 1000 mg a day.

MENSTRUAL CRAMP RELIEF: HERBAL REMEDIES FOR COMFORT

Relaxing the uterine muscles and reducing inflammation can provide much-needed relief from menstrual discomfort, and certain herbs naturally support this process.

GINGER AND CINNAMON INFUSION

A warming blend that improves circulation and reduces cramps.

Ingredients

- ½ tsp grated ginger
- ½ tsp cinnamon
- 1 cup hot water
- honey to taste (optional)

Instructions

- Place the ginger and cinnamon in a teapot and pour hot water over. Cover and steep for 10 minutes. Drink up to three times daily during your period. Do not use this remedy longer than a week.

CRAMP BARK DECOCTION

Relaxes uterine muscles and eases spasms.

Ingredients

- 1 tsp dried cramp bark
- 1 cup water

Instructions

- In a small saucepan, bring water to a boil. Lower the heat to a simmer and add the cramp bark. Simmer for 15 minutes. Strain and drink as needed. Cramp bark has a rich and fruity taste, but feel free to sweeten the remedy with honey if needed.

CHAMOMILE AND LAVENDER COMPRESS

Relaxes abdominal muscles and relieves cramping.

Ingredients

- 1 tbsp dried chamomile
- 1 tbsp dried lavender
- 2 cups hot water

Instructions

- Place the herbs in a teapot or cup. Cover and steep the herbs for 10 minutes. Afterwards, strain the liquid into a bowl. Soak a cloth in the tea and apply to the lower abdomen. Keep the compress in place for 20 minutes and repeat the treatment as needed.

MENOPAUSE AND PERIMENOPAUSE: HERBAL INFUSIONS FOR HORMONAL SHIFTS

Hot flashes, night sweats, and mood swings can be challenging, but the right herbs offer natural relief and support hormonal balance.

BLACK COHOSH TEA

Traditionally used to support estrogen balance and reduce hot flashes.

Ingredients

- 1 tsp dried black cohosh root
- 1 cup hot water

Instructions

- Place the herb in a cup or teapot. Pour hot water over and steep covered for 10–15 minutes, strain, and drink daily.

SAGE AND PEPPERMINT COOLING TEA

Reduces excessive sweating and hot flashes.

Ingredients

- 1 tsp dried sage
- 1 tsp dried peppermint
- 1 cup hot water

Instructions

- Steep the herbs in a covered teapot or cup for 10 minutes, strain, and drink as needed. Avoid this remedy if you are allergic to the mint family, or if mint-based remedies give you headaches.

RED CLOVER INFUSION

Contains phytoestrogens that may support hormonal transitions.

Ingredients

- 1 tbsp dried red clover
- 1 cup hot water

Instructions

- Steep the herb in a covered teapot for 15 minutes. Drink daily in the mid-morning or afternoon. If you plan to drink this tea for more than three months, take a one-week break each month to ensure safe and effective use of the herb.

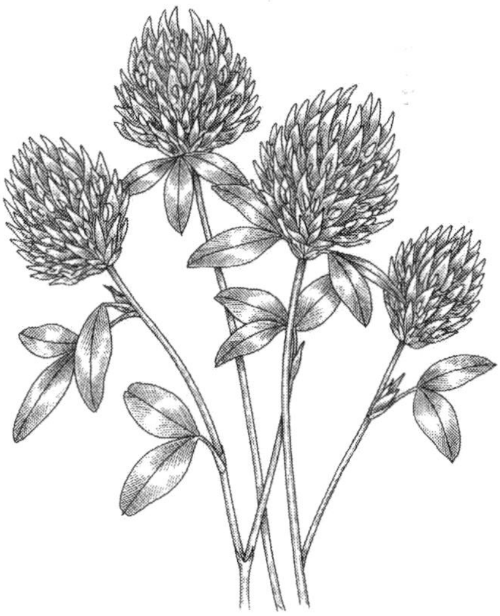

FERTILITY BOOSTING TONIC: HERBAL SUPPORT FOR CONCEPTION

Nourishing the reproductive system and supporting fertility, these herbs help promote overall reproductive health.

MACA ROOT AND ASHWAGANDHA INFUSION

Supports hormone balance and energy levels.

Ingredients

- 1 tsp dried maca root powder
- 1 tsp dried ashwagandha root (or ½ tsp powdered ashwagandha)
- 1 cup hot water
- honey (optional)

Instructions

- Add maca root and ashwagandha to a heatproof jar or teapot. Pour hot (not boiling) water over the herbs. Cover and steep for 10–15 minutes. Strain and sweeten with honey if preferred. Drink once or twice daily for best results. After three months of continuous use, take a break for two weeks before resuming.

RED RASPBERRY AND NETTLE INFUSION

Rich in minerals that support fertility.

Ingredients

- 1 tbsp dried red raspberry leaf
- 1 tbsp dried nettle leaf
- 2 cups hot water
- Lemon or honey (optional)

Instructions

- Place the dried herbs in a teapot. Pour hot water over the herbs and cover. Steep for 20–30 minutes (or longer for a stronger infusion). Strain and add honey or lemon to enhance the flavor profile. Drink warm or enjoy as an iced tea. It is advisable not to drink more than two cups a day. If you plan to use this remedy continuously for several months, take a week-long break every three months for safety reasons.

DONG QUAI AND SHATAVARI TINCTURE

Traditionally used to balance hormones and promote circulation to reproductive organs.

Ingredients

- 1 cup dried dong quai root
- 1 cup dried shatavari root
- 4 cups 80-proof alcohol (vodka or brandy)

Instructions

- Place the herbs in a clean glass jar. Pour alcohol over until fully submerged, leaving an inch of space at the top. Seal the jar and store it away from sources of direct light and heat (like a cupboard) for six weeks. Strain the tincture into a clean bottle and store in a dark glass dropper bottle. Take 30–40 drops (about one dropperful) in water or tea once or twice daily. After three months of continuous use, take a two-week break before resuming to ensure safe and effective use.

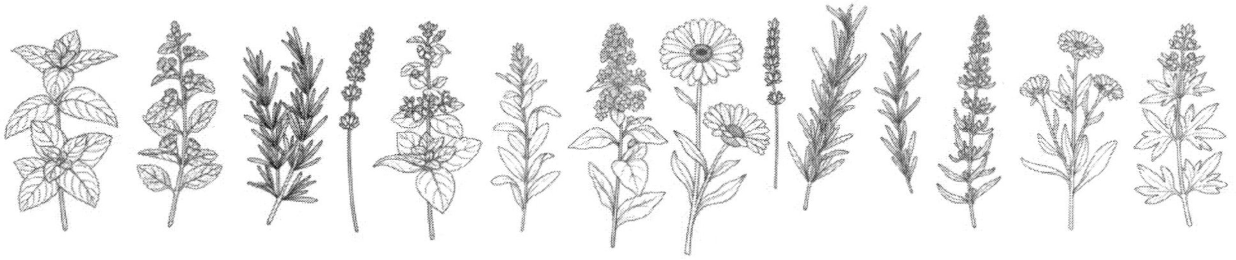

NATURE'S APHRODISIAC: HERBAL BLENDS FOR LIBIDO AND PASSION

These herbal blends are crafted to boost libido, improve circulation, and support hormonal vitality – giving your body a little extra spark when things get steamy.

DAMIANA AND MUIRA PUAMA INFUSION

Boosts libido and energy.

Ingredients

- 1 tsp dried damiana leaf
- 1 tsp dried muira puama bark
- 1 cup hot water
- honey or lemon (optional)

Instructions

- Place damiana and muira puama in a heatproof teapot. Pour hot (not boiling) water over and steep covered for 10–15 minutes. Strain the herbs and sweeten with honey or add lemon if desired. Drink up to twice a day for enhanced vitality. If pregnant, breastfeeding, or on hormone-related medications, consult a healthcare professional before use.

CACAO ADAPTOGEN TONIC

Supports stamina, hormone balance, and desire.

Ingredients

- 1 tsp maca root powder
- 1 tsp raw cacao powder
- 1 cup warm water or almond milk
- 1 tsp honey (optional)

Instructions

- Mix maca root powder and raw cacao powder into warm water or almond milk. Stir until well combined. Sweeten with honey if you like. Drink once daily to support stamina and balance hormones. It's not advisable to drink more than one cup every day. This remedy can be used consistently for up to three months. Thereafter, take a two-week break before resuming use. If you have a sensitive stomach or caffeine intolerance, start with a smaller dose or avoid the remedy altogether.

ROSE AND CINNAMON HERBAL ELIXIR

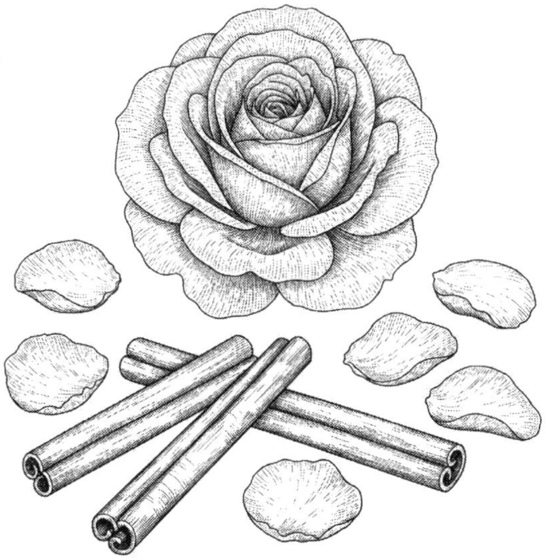

Stimulates the senses and warms circulation.

Ingredients

- 1 tbsp dried rose petals
- 1 tsp ground cinnamon
- 1 cup hot water
- 1-2 tsp honey or maple syrup (optional)

Instructions

- Add dried rose petals and ground cinnamon to a teapot. Pour hot water over the herbs and cover. Steep for 10–15 minutes. Strain and sweeten with honey or maple syrup if desired. Drink once a day. Rose and cinnamon are safe for long-term use, but it's best to take breaks (at least one week) after three months to ensure safety. If you have cinnamon sensitivity or are pregnant, consult a healthcare provider before use.

PCOS AND HORMONAL ACNE: HERBAL REMEDIES FOR ANDROGEN BALANCE

When hormones go haywire, it can lead to stubborn acne, irregular cycles, and other frustrating PCOS symptoms. Fortunately, certain herbs can help bring balance, supporting healthy androgen levels and promoting clearer skin from the inside out.

SPEARMINT TEA

May help lower elevated testosterone levels.

For detailed brewing instructions, see *Menstrual Cycle Support: Herbal Teas for Balance.*

LICORICE ROOT AND WHITE PEONY INFUSION

Supports ovarian health and hormone regulation.

Ingredients

- 1 tsp dried licorice root
- 1 tsp dried white peony root
- 1 ½ cups hot water

Instructions

- Add the dried herbs to a heatproof mug or teapot. Pour hot water over the herbs and steep for 10–15 minutes. Strain and drink once daily for hormonal support. This remedy can be used daily for up to three months; thereafter, take a month-long break before resuming use. If you live with high blood pressure or are taking medications to manage blood pressure, it is best to avoid this remedy. Best taken in the morning or early afternoon to avoid affecting sleep.

BURDOCK ROOT TINCTURE

Aids liver detox to clear excess hormones contributing to acne.

Ingredients

- 1 cup dried burdock root
- 2 cups high-proof alcohol (vodka or brandy)

Instructions

- Place the dried burdock root in a glass jar. Submerge the herbs with alcohol.. Seal the jar tightly and store it in a cool, dark place for six weeks, shaking occasionally. After steeping, strain through a cheesecloth into a dark glass dropper bottle. Take 30 to 40 drops (about half a teaspoon) in water or tea, up to twice daily. Safe for long-term use, but take a week-long break every six weeks. If you are allergic to the ragweed family, it is best to avoid this remedy.

HERBAL BATHS FOR HORMONAL RELAXATION AND REPRODUCTIVE SUPPORT

A warm bath is more than just a moment of self-care – it can be a powerful way to support your hormonal health. Infused with the right herbs, a soak can help ease menstrual cramps, boost circulation, and promote deep relaxation, giving your body the gentle support it needs.

ROSE AND LAVENDER HERBAL BATH

Promotes emotional balance and self-care.

Ingredients

- ½ cup dried rose petals
- ½ cup dried lavender buds
- 1 cup Epsom salt
- 2 tbsp carrier oil (like almond or jojoba)
- 5–10 drops lavender essential oil (optional)
- 5–10 drops rose essential oil (optional)

Instructions

- Mix the dried herbs and Epsom salt in a bowl. Add the carrier oil and essential oils, stirring well. Place the herbal mixture in a muslin bag or cheesecloth, securing it tightly. Drop the bag into a warm bath and let it infuse for 5–10 minutes before soaking. Soak for 20–30 minutes to absorb the calming herbal properties.

GINGER AND CHAMOMILE WARM SOAK

Reduces cramps and muscle tension.

Ingredients

- 5-10 drops ginger essential oil (optional)
- ½ cup dried chamomile flowers
- 5-10 drops chamomile essential oil (optional)
- 1 cup Epsom salt
- ¼ cup grated fresh ginger (or 2 tbsp dried ginger)

Instructions

- If using fresh ginger, place it in a pot with 2 cups of water, simmer for 10 minutes. Strain before adding to the bath. Add chamomile, Epsom salt, and essential oils directly to the bath or place in a muslin bag. Fill the tub with warm water and let the herbs steep for 5–10 minutes. Soak for 20–30 minutes, allowing the warmth to relax muscles and ease cramps.

CLARY SAGE AND LEMON BALM HORMONE-BALANCING BATH

Encourages hormonal balance and relieves stress-related tension.

Ingredients

- ½ cup dried lemon balm
- ¼ cup dried clary sage
- 1 cup Epsom salt
- 5 drops clary sage essential oil
- 5 drops lemon balm essential oil

Instructions

- Mix all ingredients in a bowl, stirring well. Place the mixture in a muslin bag and drop into a warm bath. Let the herbs steep for 10 minutes. Soak for 20–30 minutes, breathing deeply for relaxation.

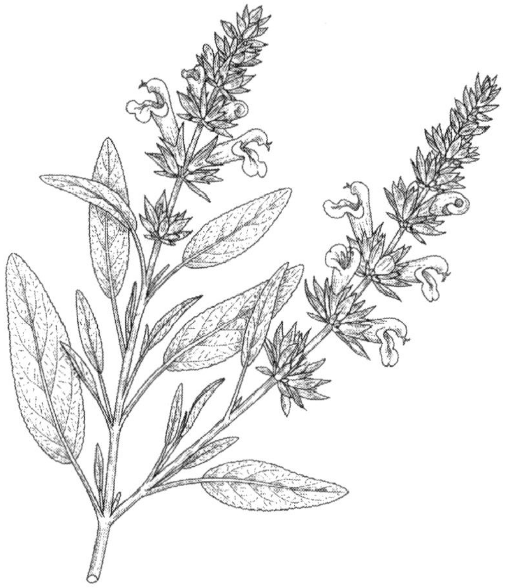

MUGWORT AND YARROW BATH

Traditionally used for uterine support and menstrual balance.

Ingredients

- ½ cup dried mugwort
- ½ cup dried yarrow
- 4 cups hot water

Instructions

- Place the dried herbs in a large heatproof bowl. Allow the herbs to steep in boiling water for at least 5 minutes. Strain and pour the infusion into a warm bath. Soak for 15–20 minutes. Use this remedy one or two times per month, avoiding use during pregnancy.

WILD YAM AND BASIL BATH

Can encourage menstrual balance, ease cramps, and promote circulation.

Ingredients

- ½ cup dried wild yam root
- ¼ cup dried basil leaves
- 1 cup Epsom salt
- 5 drops geranium essential oil (optional)

Instructions

- Add wild yam root and basil leaves to a muslin bag. Mix the essential oil with the Epsom salt and add this to the bag as well. Fill your bathtub with warm water and drop in the herbal bag. Let it steep for 5–10 minutes before getting in. Soak for 20–30 minutes.

SEED CYCLING FOR HORMONAL BALANCE

Seed cycling is a natural way to help balance hormones during the menstrual cycle by eating different seeds at different times. The aim is to support the two main hormones, estrogen and progesterone, as their levels change throughout the month.

Phase	Days	Seeds to use	Seed benefits	How to use
Follicular Phase	Days 1-14	Flaxseeds and pumpkin seeds	*Flaxseeds:* Rich in lignans to help balance estrogen levels. *Pumpkin seeds:* High in zinc to support hormone production.	Ground up to two tablespoons of each and add to smoothies, yogurt, or salads.
Luteal Phase	Days 15-28	Sunflower and sesame seeds	*Sunflower seeds*: Rich in Vitamin E to support progesterone. *Sesame seeds*: Contain lignans to balance progesterone.	Ground up to two tablespoons of each and sprinkle on salads, add to smoothies, or bake into goods.

During the Follicular Phase (Days 1-14), starting from the first day of your period until ovulation, your body increases estrogen. Eating flaxseeds and pumpkin seeds helps during this time. Flaxseeds have nutrients that support healthy estrogen processing, while pumpkin seeds are high in zinc, which helps hormone production and keeps estrogen levels stable. You can add 1–2 tablespoons of ground flaxseeds and pumpkin seeds to smoothies, yogurt, salads, or oatmeal, making sure the flaxseeds are ground for better use by your body. These seeds also have fiber, which helps remove extra estrogen.

In the Luteal Phase (Days 15-28), after ovulation, your body needs more progesterone in case of pregnancy or the start of your next period. Sunflower seeds and sesame seeds are good options during this phase. Sunflower seeds are rich in vitamin E, which helps maintain progesterone levels and aids ovarian function necessary for producing progesterone. Sesame seeds also contain nutrients that help balance progesterone. Like in the follicular phase, you can add 1–2 tablespoons of ground sunflower seeds and sesame seeds to your meals, such as in smoothies, salads, or baked goods.

Seed cycling is based on the idea that different phases of the menstrual cycle need different hormonal support. When we eat the right seeds at the right time, your body gets the nutrients it needs to balance estrogen and progesterone naturally. This may help reduce symptoms like cramps, acne, and mood swings and lead to a more regular cycle.

To see the benefits of seed cycling, it's best to try it for at least three months (Kovacevic, 2024). It may take a few cycles for your body to adjust and for the seeds to show their full effect.

If you don't like the taste of seeds, you can easily add them to your diet by blending them into smoothies or baking them into muffins or energy balls. Ground flaxseeds have a mild taste when mixed with food.

CHAPTER 12:

BRAIN AND NERVE HEALTH

Your brain and nervous system do a lot – they keep your memory sharp, help you stay focused, balance your mood, and keep you feeling your best. In this chapter, we'll explore herbal and natural remedies that support brain function, emotional well-being, and nerve health. Whether you're looking to boost memory, clear brain fog, ease nerve pain, or just give your nervous system some extra love, these remedies can help you feel sharper and more balanced every day.

MEMORY ENHANCEMENT: HERBAL TEAS AND TONICS

Boost your memory and mental clarity with herbal teas and tonics that improve circulation and protect against oxidative stress. These natural remedies help keep your brain sharp and focused.

GINKGO BILOBA TEA

Improves blood flow to the brain and enhances memory.

Ingredients

- 1 tsp dried Ginkgo Biloba leaves
- 1 cup hot water

Instructions

- Boil water and pour it over the herb. For the next 10 minutes leave the herbs to steep while covered. Strain the tea and discard the leaves. Drink once daily.

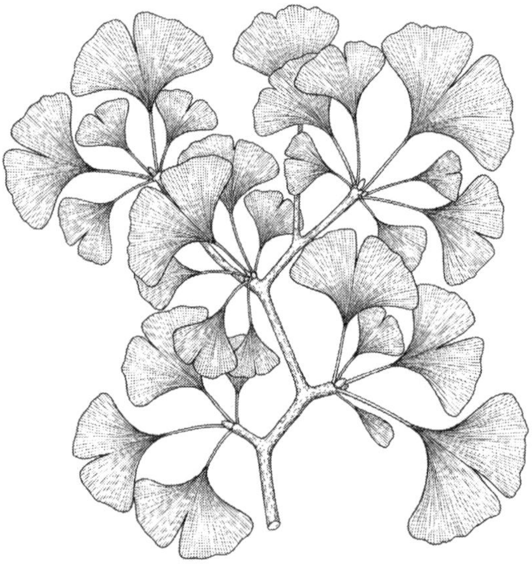

BACOPA MONNIERI TINCTURE

Supports cognitive function and mental clarity.

Ingredients

- 1 ounce of Dried Bacopa Monnieri (you can find this at health food stores or online)
- 2 cups of high-proof alcohol (such as vodka or brandy; at least 40-50% alcohol by volume)
- A clean glass jar with a tight-fitting lid

Instructions

- Chop or grind the herb slightly to increase its surface area. Place in a clean glass jar. Pour enough alcohol over the herb to fully submerge it. Close the jar tightly with a lid to prevent evaporation and contamination. Store in a cool, dark place for four weeks. Shake the jar gently every other day to help the extraction process. Strain the tincture and transfer into an amber container. Keep it in a cool, dark place. To use, take 30 drops of the tincture in water, once or twice daily.

ROSEMARY INFUSION

Boosts concentration and mental alertness.

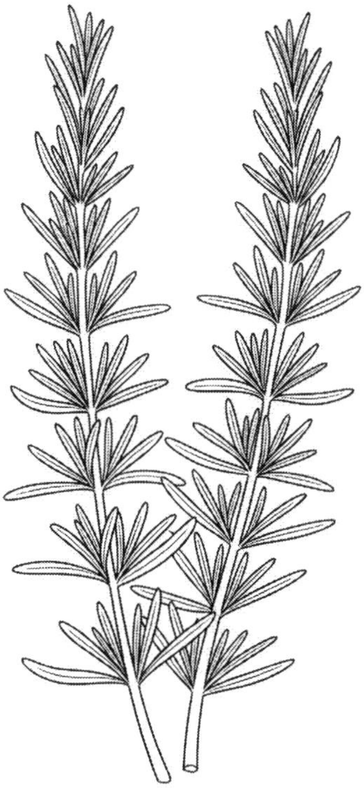

Ingredients

- fresh rosemary (about 1-2 sprigs)
- 2 cups of hot water

Instructions

- Boil water and pour it over the fresh rosemary sprigs in a teapot. Cover and let it steep for 10 minutes. Strain the infusion and discard the spent herbs. Drink up to twice daily for enhanced concentration and alertness.

NEUROPROTECTION: HERBAL REMEDIES FOR NERVE HEALTH

Keep your nervous system strong with herbal remedies that protect neurons and support long-term brain health. Natural solutions can help maintain cognitive function and overall well-being.

GOLDEN MILK

Reduces brain inflammation and supports cognitive longevity.

For detailed brewing instructions, see Chapter Nine, *Joint Pain: Herbal Remedies for Arthritis Relief.*

ASHWAGANDHA TINCTURE

Reduces oxidative stress and improves brain resilience.

Ingredients

- 1 ounce of dried Ashwagandha root
- 2 cups of high-proof alcohol
- a clean glass jar with a tight-fitting lid

Instructions

- Chop or grind the herb slightly and place it in a glass jar. Pour enough alcohol over the root to fully cover it. Seal the jar tightly and store in a cool, dark place for six weeks. Shake the jar gently every second day to aid extraction. Strain the tincture through a fine-mesh strainer or cheesecloth into a clean bottle or jar. Discard the spent herbs and store the tincture in an amber dropper bottle for easy use. Keep it in a cool, dark place. To use, take 30 drops once a day in water.

GOTU KOLA TEA

Enhances nerve regeneration and cognitive function.

Ingredients

- 1 tsp dried Gotu Kola leaves (or 1-2 fresh leaves)
- 1 cup hot water

Instructions

- Boil water and pour it over the dried or fresh Gotu Kola leaves in a teapot or tea infuser. The tea should be allowed to steep for 5-10 minutes. Strain the leaves and discard them. Drink once daily to support cognitive function and nerve health.

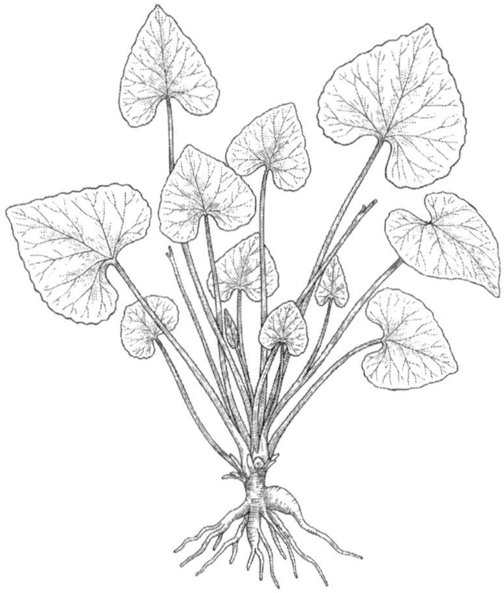

MOOD ENHANCEMENT: HERBAL REMEDIES FOR EMOTIONAL WELL-BEING

Lift your spirits and find balance with herbs that support mood stability and emotional resilience.

ST. JOHN'S WORT TEA

Supports mood balance and mild depression relief.

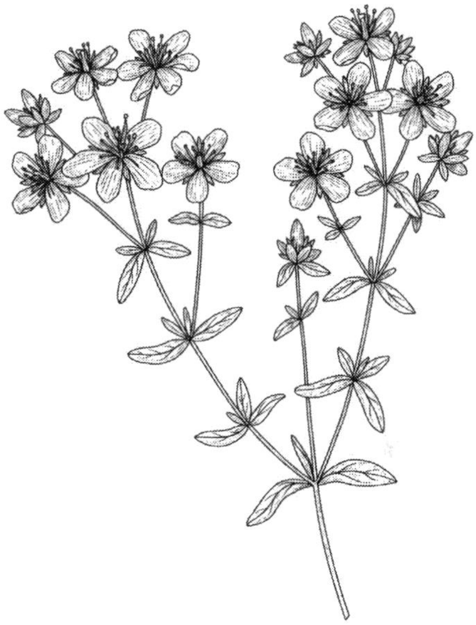

Ingredients

- 1 tsp dried St. John's Wort
- 1 cup hot water

Instructions

- Heat water until just below a boil. Pour over the dried herb, cover, and steep for 5–10 minutes. Strain and drink once daily, preferably in the morning or early afternoon, with meals to avoid stomach irritation.
- This tea is most effective for mild to moderate low mood and emotional stress, with benefits building over two to four weeks of consistent use. It can be taken for up to three months, after which a break of at least one week is recommended. To minimize potential side effects, consider gradually reducing the strength and frequency of the tea in the week leading up to your break.
- St. John's Wort interacts with several medications and may cause photosensitivity – consult a healthcare provider before use.

SAFFRON INFUSION

Naturally uplifts mood and reduces symptoms of depression.

Ingredients

- 3-5 saffron threads
- 1 cup hot water
- ½ tsp honey for sweetness
- two or three fresh mint sprigs (optional, to enhance taste and combat nausea)

Instructions

- Heat water until warm but not boiling. Add three to five saffron threads (and mint if using) and let them steep for 10–15 minutes. Stir and enjoy once daily: Use daily for four to six weeks to see consistent benefits. Avoid high doses, as excessive saffron can cause dizziness or nausea.

DAMIANA LEAF TEA

Promotes relaxation and eases emotional tension.

Ingredients

- 1 tsp dried Damiana leaves
- 1 cup hot water
- ½ tsp honey or lemon (optional, to enhance taste)

Instructions

- Bring water to a near boil. Add dried Damiana leaves. Cover and steep for 10 minutes. Strain and drink once or twice daily. Best taken in the evening or when needing emotional relaxation.

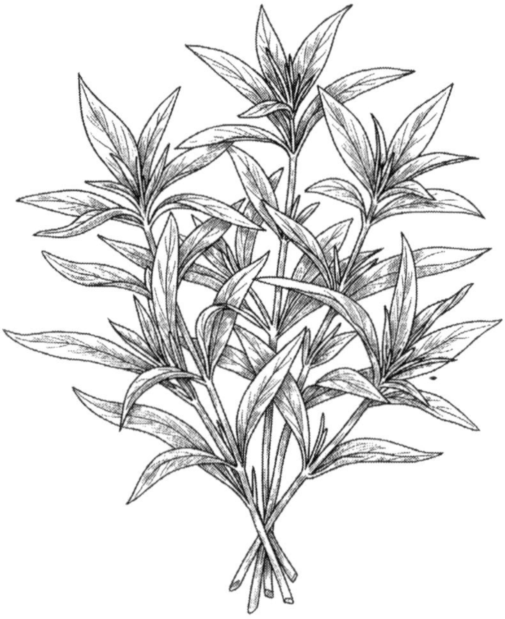

COGNITIVE FUNCTION: HERBAL REMEDIES FOR FOCUS AND CONCENTRATION

Sharpen your mind and stay focused with herbs that enhance mental clarity and reduce brain fog.

SAGE TEA

Improves cognitive function and memory recall.

Ingredients

- 1 tsp dried sage leaves (or 1-2 fresh sage leaves)
- 1 cup hot water

Instructions

- Boil water and pour it over the dried or fresh sage leaves in a teapot or tea infuser. Let the tea steep for 5-10 minutes. Strain the leaves and discard them. Drink once daily to support cognitive function and enhance memory recall.

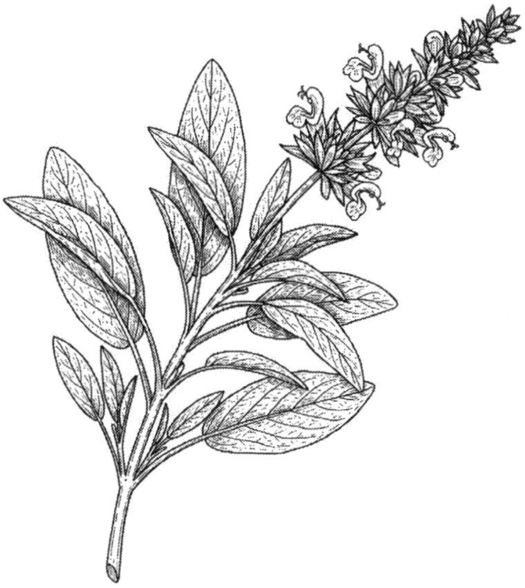

PEPPERMINT TEA

Stimulates mental alertness.

See Chapter Six, *Cold and Flu: Herbal Teas for Symptom Relief*, for detailed brewing instructions.

GINSENG TINCTURE

Increases mental performance and combats fatigue.

Ingredients

- 1 ounce of dried ginseng root
- 2 cups of high-proof alcohol
- a clean glass jar with a tight-fitting lid

Instructions

- Chop or grind the dried ginseng root slightly for better extraction. Place the herb in the glass jar and pour alcohol over, ensuring it is completely submerged. Use a cupboard or any other cool, dark place to store the jar for a maximum of six weeks. Thereafter, strain the extract through a fine-mesh strainer or cheesecloth into a clean bottle and transfer into a dark glass bottle with a dropper. Keep it in a cool, dark place. Take 30-40 drops in water once or twice daily, preferably in the morning or early afternoon.

BRAIN FOG: HERBAL REMEDIES FOR MENTAL CLARITY

Clear the fog and boost your focus with herbs that help sharpen your mind and reduce sluggish thinking.

GOTU KOLA INFUSION

Enhances clarity and processing speed.

Ingredients

- 1 tsp dried Gotu Kola leaves
- 1 cup hot water

Instructions

- Heat water until just below a boil. Pour over Gotu Kola leaves, cover, and steep for 10 minutes. Strain and drink once daily for sustained cognitive benefits. Best used in cycles lasting four to six weeks with a one-week break to prevent potential side effects.

LEMON BALM TEA

Reduces stress-induced brain fog and improves concentration.

For detailed brewing instructions, see Chapter 10, *Anxiety: Herbal Remedies for Calming the Mind.*

GINKGO BILOBA TINCTURE

Increases oxygen flow to the brain and sharpens focus.

Ingredients

- 1 ounce dried Ginkgo Biloba leaves
- 2 cups high-proof alcohol
- a clean glass jar with a tight-fitting lid

Instructions

- Lightly crush the dried Ginkgo Biloba leaves for better extraction. Place the leaves in the glass jar and pour alcohol over them, ensuring they are fully submerged. A cool, dark place without direct light and heat sources is ideal to store the jar for six weeks, shaking occasionally. Use a cheesecloth or a fine-mesh strainer to strain the liquid. Transfer into a dark glass dropper bottle and store in a cool, dark place. Take 30 drops in water once or twice daily, preferably in the morning or early afternoon.

PARKINSON'S AND NEURODEGENERATIVE SUPPORT: HERBAL REMEDIES FOR NERVOUS SYSTEM PROTECTION

Support your nervous system with herbs that protect neurons, slow degeneration, and help maintain motor function.

GOLDEN MILK

Reduces neuroinflammation and protects against oxidative stress.

For detailed brewing instructions, see Chapter Nine, *Joint Pain: Herbal Remedies for Arthritis Relief.*

LION'S MANE MUSHROOM TEA

Supports nerve regeneration and brain health.

Ingredients

- 1 tablespoon dried Lion's Mane mushroom (or 2 tablespoons fresh)
- 2 cups water

Instructions

- Bring water to a boil, then reduce to a simmer. Add the Lion's Mane mushroom and let it simmer for 20–30 minutes. Strain and drink once or twice daily. Add honey or lemon for taste. Lion's Mane is best consumed consistently for at least four to six weeks for noticeable cognitive benefits.

GREEN TEA EXTRACT

Prevents cognitive decline and promotes longevity.

Ingredients

- 1 ounce (about 2 tablespoons) high-quality green tea leaves
- 2 cups high-proof alcohol
- a clean glass jar with a tight-fitting lid

Instructions

- Lightly crush the green tea leaves to increase surface area. Place the leaves in a clean glass jar and pour the alcohol over them, ensuring they are fully submerged. For six weeks, keep the jar hidden in a cupboard or any other cool, dark place where direct light and heat sources won't be a factor, shaking occasionally. Strain the liquid through a fine-mesh strainer or cheesecloth into a clean container and transfer into a dark glass dropper bottle for storage. Take 30–40 drops in water or tea once or twice daily. Best taken in the morning or early afternoon due to caffeine content.

CHAPTER 13:

FACE, HAIR, AND PERSONAL CARE

Cleopatra's legendary beauty wasn't just a myth – it was the result of carefully crafted natural rituals. From her famous milk and honey baths to herbal-infused oils, she understood the power of plants in enhancing skin, hair, and overall well-being. Today, we can take a page from her book by harnessing the benefits of herbal and natural remedies to nourish our skin, strengthen our hair, and elevate personal care – all without the harsh synthetic chemicals found in modern products. With the wisdom of ancient traditions and the science of plant-based ingredients, you can create a beauty routine that is both luxurious and effective.

FACIAL CARE: HERBAL REMEDIES FOR CLEAR AND RADIANT SKIN

Give your skin the care it deserves with herbs that cleanse, tone, and hydrate – naturally. Whether you're dealing with acne, dryness, or dullness, these plant-powered remedies help restore balance, leaving your skin glowing and healthy.

CHAMOMILE FACIAL STEAM

Opens pores and soothes irritated skin.

Ingredients

- 1 tbsp dried chamomile flowers
- 4 cups of boiling water
- big bowl

Instructions

- Add dried chamomile flowers to a bowl of boiling water. Drape a towel over your head and let the steam gently cleanse your face for 5–10 minutes. Suitable for all skin types. Use a maximum of two times a week to reduce redness, calm inflammation, and open pores. After steaming, pat the face dry with a soft towel, tone, and moisturize.

ALOE VERA MOISTURIZER

Hydrates the skin and reduces redness.

Ingredients

- 1 tsp of aloe vera gel

Instructions

- Apply fresh aloe vera gel to your face daily after cleansing and toning. Aloe vera is suitable for all skin types.

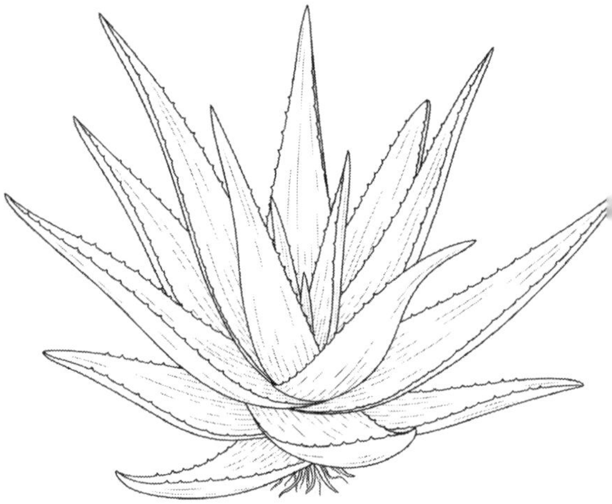

CALENDULA TONER

Reduces inflammation and promotes healing.

Ingredients

- 1 cup of calendula flowers (fresh or dried)
- 4 cups of witch hazel
- glass jar

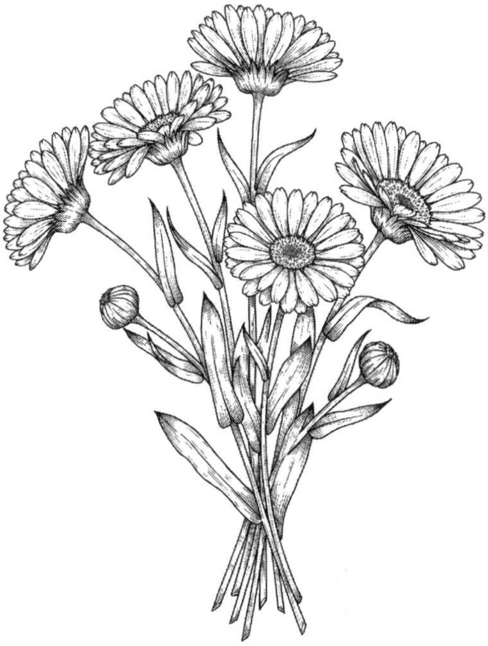

Instructions

- Place the calendula flowers in a glass jar and pour witch hazel over. Ensure the flowers are completely submerged and seal the jar tightly. Store in a cool, dark place. Allow the mixture to infuse for one week, then strain into a clean container and use as a toner after cleansing. This toner is safe to use on all skin types.

HAIR CARE: HERBAL TREATMENTS FOR STRONG AND SHINY HAIR

Nourish your hair from root to tip with herbal remedies that strengthen follicles, boost growth, and keep dandruff at bay. These natural treatments help you achieve healthier, shinier hair – without the harsh chemicals.

ROSEMARY HAIR RINSE

Stimulates hair growth and adds shine.

Ingredients

- 2 tbsp dried rosemary (or two sprigs of fresh rosemary)
- 2 cups of boiling water

Instructions

- Create a strong infusion by allowing the rosemary to steep in boiling hot water until cool. Strain the mixture and use it to rinse your hair (works best when used as a final hair rinse). Rosemary will not only leave your hair shiny, but the uplifting aroma will help to alleviate mental fatigue. Consistent use may cause the hair to turn slightly darker.

NETTLE INFUSION

Nourishes the scalp and reduces dandruff.

Ingredients

- 2 tbsp dried nettle leaves
- 2 cups of boiling water

Instructions

- Steep nettle leaves in boiling water until cooled. Stain and use as a scalp rinse. This extra-strong infusion is intended for external use only.

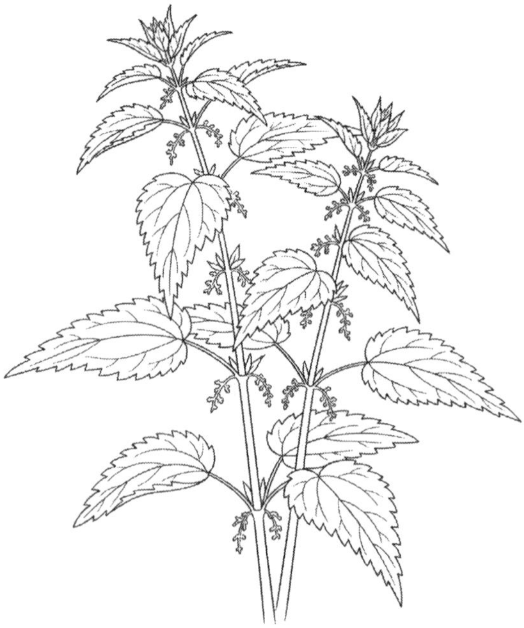

HIBISCUS HAIR MASK

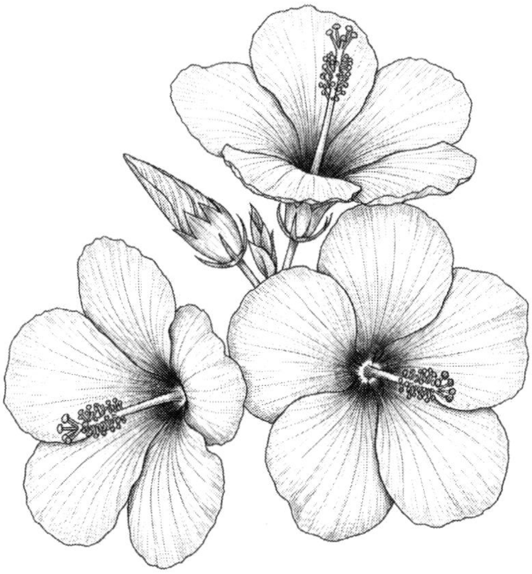

Conditions hair and prevents premature graying.

Ingredients

- half a cup of dried hibiscus flowers
- enough water to form a paste

Instructions

- Grind hibiscus petals into a paste with water. Apply to hair, focusing on the scalp and spreading it evenly over the strands. Leave the hair mask on for half an hour, and afterwards rinse it out using warm water. This remedy is suitable for all hair types and can be used up to two times a week to combat premature greying, restore strength, and balance oil production. For an extra nourishing mask, mix in some jojoba or argan oil into the paste and apply to the hair. This is an excellent option if the hair is very dry and damaged.

LIP CARE: HERBAL REMEDIES FOR SOFT AND SUPPLE LIPS

Say goodbye to dry, chapped lips! These natural ingredients deeply moisturize, heal, and protect, leaving your lips soft, smooth, and healthy.

BEESWAX AND HONEY LIP BALM

Hydrates and protects lips.

Ingredients

- 1 tbsp beeswax
- 1 tbsp honey
- 2 tbsp coconut oil
- 1 tsp vitamin E oil

Instructions

- Melt the beeswax and stir in the honey and coconut oil. Add the vitamin E oil and stir gently until everything is incorporated. Pour the liquid into a container and let it cool before use.

PEPPERMINT LIP SCRUB

Exfoliates and invigorates lips.

Ingredients

- 1 tbsp sugar (or ground oatmeal)
- 1 tsp honey
- 1 drop of peppermint essential oil

Instructions

- Mix sugar, honey, and essential oil to create a rough paste. Gently rub onto lips for half a minute and rinse. Sugar may leave a sticky residue on the skin, so feel free to substitute it with ground oatmeal to create a gentle and effective scrub that's safe for all skin types.

CALENDULA INFUSED OIL

Heals cracked lips.

For detailed instructions on how to make this oil, see Chapter Eight, *Acne: Herbal Treatments for Clear Skin*.

ORAL CARE: HERBAL SOLUTIONS FOR FRESH BREATH AND HEALTHY GUMS

Keep your smile bright and your breath fresh with herbal remedies that support oral hygiene, promote healthy gums, and naturally freshen your breath.

SAGE MOUTHWASH

Cleanses the mouth and freshens breath.

Ingredients

- 1 tbsp dried sage
- 1 cup of hot water

Instructions

- Steep sage in hot water until cooled. Strain and use as a mouthwash. Do not swallow this extra-strong infusion.

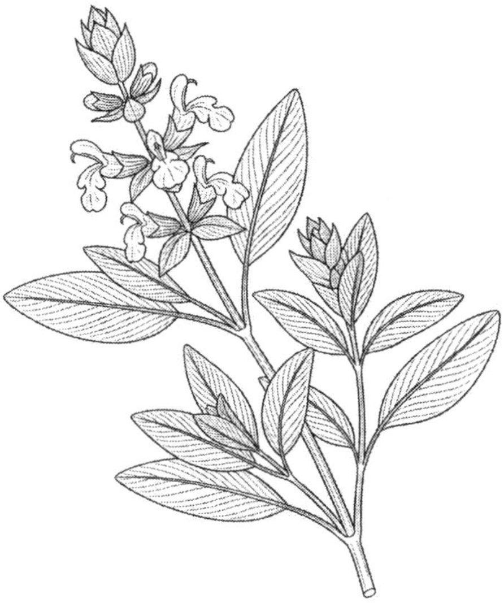

CLOVE OIL TOOTHPASTE

Reduces bacteria and soothes toothaches.

Instructions

- I2 tbsp coconut oil (antibacterial base)
- 1 tbsp baking soda (cleans and whitens teeth)
- two drops clove essential oil (reduces bacteria and soothes pain)

Instructions

- In a small bowl, mix coconut oil and baking soda until smooth. Add clove oil and stir well. Store in an airtight container. To use, scoop a small amount onto your toothbrush and brush as usual. If the mixture is too solid, slightly warm the coconut oil before mixing. Use once or twice daily for best results.

MYRRH GUM POWDER

Prevents gum inflammation.

Ingredients

Myrrh resin chunks (dried) – 1 tbsp, or desired amount

Instructions

- Place the myrrh resin chunks in the freezer for two hours. This makes them more brittle and easier to grind. Use a mortar and pestle to crush the resin into a fine powder. Alternatively, you can use a spice grinder for a smooth, fine texture. If you want an ultra-fine powder, sift it through a fine-mesh sieve and regrind any larger particles. Store the powder in an airtight container, sealing out any moisture. Keep the container in a cool and dry place, away from direct sources of heat and moisture. To use, simply massage a small amount onto the gums. You can also mix the powered with coconut oil or lukewarm water to form a paste and use as a natural gum treatment.

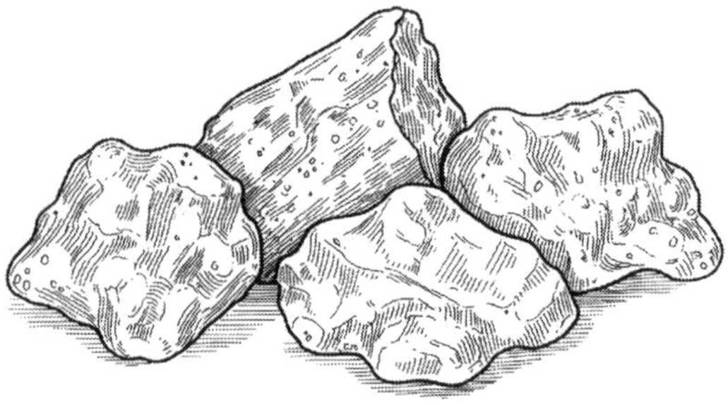

HAND AND FOOT CARE: HERBAL TREATMENTS FOR SOFT SKIN AND NAIL HEALTH

Pamper your hands and feet with herbal remedies that soften rough skin, heal cracks, and strengthen nails, leaving your skin feeling smooth and your nails looking healthy.

LAVENDER HAND SOAK

Relaxes muscles and softens skin.

Ingredients

- 5-10 drops of lavender essential oil
- 1 tbsp of carrier oil (Argan, jojoba, or avocado works well)

Instructions

- Mix lavender essential oil with carrier oil and pour into a small basin filled with warm water. Give your hands a 10-minute soak, then pat them dry. Moisturize with jojoba oil for an extra soft, non-greasy feel.

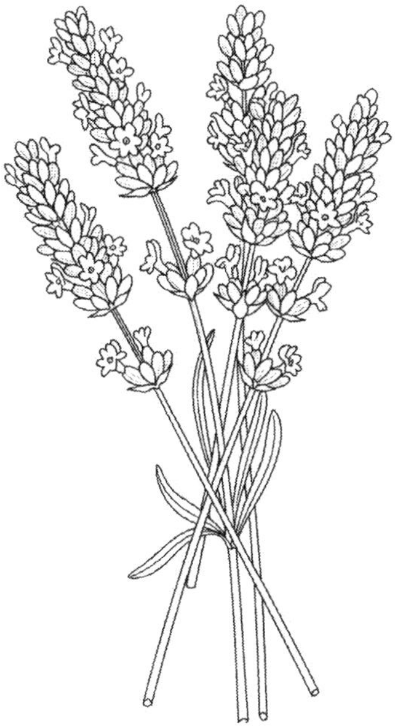

HORSETAIL NAIL STRENGTHENER

Enhances nail strength and prevents brittleness.

Ingredients

- 1 tbsp dried horsetail herb
- 1 cup boiling water

Instructions

Steep the dried horsetail in boiling water for 10–15 minutes to create a strong tea. Let it cool slightly until it's warm but comfortable to touch. Soak your nails in the tea for 10 minutes, then pat them dry. Finish by applying a natural moisturizer or cuticle oil. For weak and brittle nails, use this remedy up to three times a week. For general nail maintenance and health, use once a week.

PEPPERMINT FOOT SCRUB

Exfoliates and refreshes tired feet.

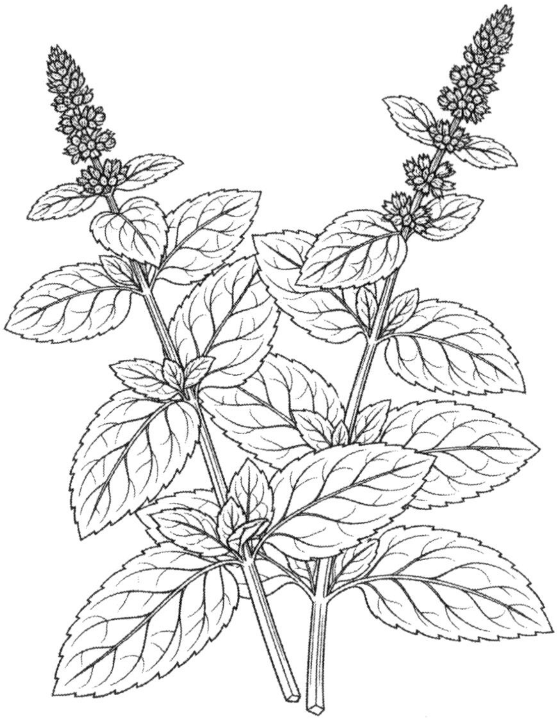

Ingredients

- half a cup of sea salt
- a quarter cup of olive oil
- 5 drops of peppermint essential oil
- 2 drops of wintergreen essential oil (optional, but enhances the cooling effect)

Instructions

- Mix the essential oils and olive oil until fully combined. Pour the oil into a bowl with salt and stir. You want a add just enough oil to create a grainy, clumpy texture. For best results, soften the skin on your feet first by soaking for five minutes in lukewarm water. Pat dry and apply the scrub in small, circular motions. Focus on areas where skin tends to be dry and cracked.

BODY CARE: HERBAL REMEDIES FOR SMOOTH AND HYDRATED SKIN

Treat your skin to natural ingredients that exfoliate, hydrate, and tone, leaving your body feeling soft, smooth, and deeply moisturized.

OATMEAL AND HONEY BODY SCRUB

Gently exfoliates and hydrates the skin.

Ingredients

- I cup ground oatmeal
- a quarter cup honey
- a quarter cup salt (optional)

Instructions

- Mix ground oatmeal with honey and gently massage onto your skin using small circular motions. This gentle scrub is safe for the face, providing a soothing exfoliation. For a deeper exfoliation, add salt to the mixture, but use it only on the body, not the face. Exfoliate once a week for smooth, refreshed skin.

GREEN TEA BATH SOAK

Detoxifies and rejuvenates the skin.

Ingredients

- Six green tea bags (or ½ cup loose green tea)

Instructions

- Fill your bathtub with warm water. Add the green tea bags directly to the water or place loose green tea in a muslin bag. Let the tea steep for 10 minutes. Soak in the bath for 15–20 minutes to detoxify and refresh your skin. Pat your skin dry and follow with a natural moisturizer if needed. Use this remedy once a week.

COCONUT AND TURMERIC BODY BUTTER

Moisturizes and brightens the skin.

Ingredients

- ½ cup coconut oil (solid or softened)
- 1 tsp turmeric powder
- 5–10 drops essential oil (optional, for fragrance)

Instructions

- In a small bowl, mix the coconut oil and turmeric powder until fully blended. Apply a small amount to your skin, massaging in circular motions until absorbed. Allow it to sit for a few minutes before dressing, as turmeric can stain fabrics. Use daily or as needed. For sensitive skin, it is best to use it two to three times a week first and check for any irritation. To prevent staining, use less turmeric or wipe off excess product after 10–15 minutes.

PERSONAL HYGIENE: HERBAL DEODORANTS AND ANTIPERSPIRANTS

Keep fresh all day with herbal deodorants that naturally neutralize body odor and help reduce perspiration – without the harsh chemicals.

WITCH HAZEL AND LAVENDER DEODORANT

Eliminates odor-causing bacteria.

Ingredients

- 2 tbsp witch hazel
- 10-15 drops lavender essential oil

Instructions

- Mix the witch hazel and lavender essential oil in a spray bottle. Shake well to combine. Spray under your arms as needed.

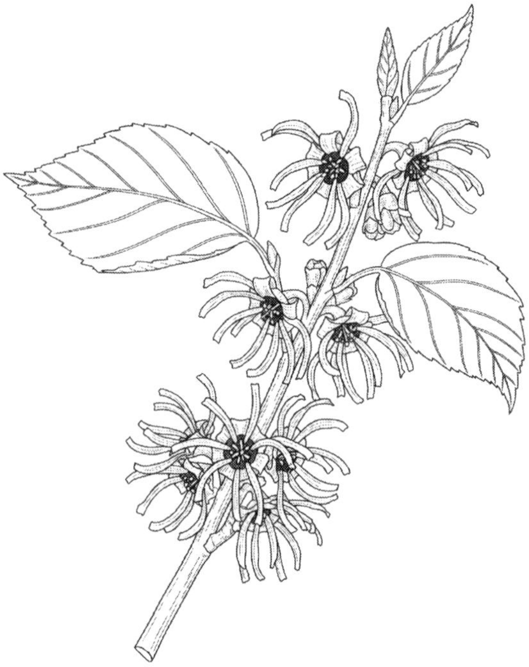

SAGE AND ROSEMARY POWDER

Absorbs moisture and prevents odor.

Ingredients

- 1 tbsp dried sage
- 1 tbsp dried rosemary

Instructions

- Grind the dried sage and rosemary into a fine powder using a mortar and pestle or a spice grinder. Gently apply the powder to your underarms to absorb moisture and prevent odor. Apply as needed.

COCONUT OIL AND BAKING SODA PASTE

Acts as a natural antiperspirant.

Ingredients

- 2 tbsp coconut oil (solid or softened)
- 2 tbsp baking soda
- 5 drops tea tree oil

Instructions

- Make a smooth paste with the coconut oil and baking soda. Then stir the tea tree oil in. Apply a thin layer of the paste to your underarms. Use as needed, but this remedy may not be suitable for sensitive skin types.

GENTLE DEODORANT FOR SENSITIVE SKIN

Ingredients

- 3 tbsp coconut oil (solid or softened)
- 2 tbsp arrowroot powder (or cornstarch)
- 1 tbsp baking soda (optional, reduce or omit for extra sensitive skin)
- 10 drops lavender essential oil (or chamomile for extra soothing)
- 5 drops geranium essential oil (optional, for a light, floral scent)

Instructions

- In a small bowl, combine the coconut oil and arrowroot powder. Stir until smooth and well mixed. If using, add the baking soda and stir well. Add the essential oils. Mix everything thoroughly and transfer to a small jar. Apply a small amount to your underarms and gently massage until absorbed. Use as needed.

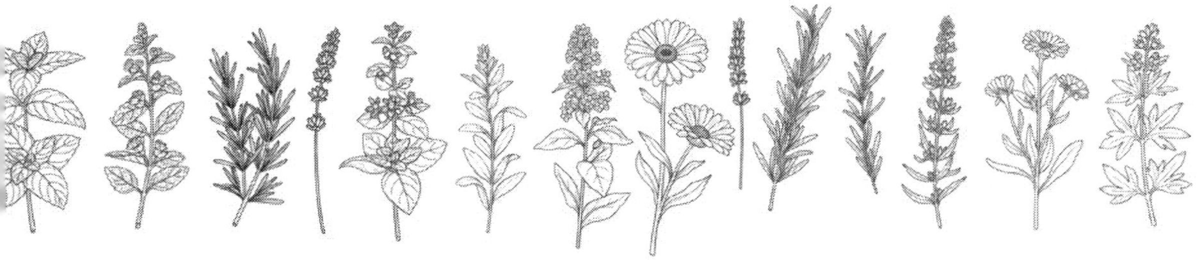

HAIR REMOVAL: NATURAL METHODS FOR REDUCING UNWANTED HAIR

Say goodbye to unwanted hair with natural ingredients that help remove hair and slow regrowth, offering a gentler alternative to modern treatments. For best results, pair these remedies with the coconut and turmeric body butter.

TURMERIC AND MILK PASTE

Weakens hair roots and slows regrowth.

Ingredients

- 1 tbsp turmeric powder
- 2 tbsp milk (or enough to form a paste)

Instructions

- Mix the turmeric powder with the milk in a small bowl. Stir until a thick paste forms. Add more milk if needed to achieve the desired consistency. Apply the paste directly onto unwanted hair and leave it on for about 15-20 minutes. Gently wipe off with a damp cloth or rinse with warm water. Apply up to three times a week for best results. Over time, this may help weaken hair roots and slow regrowth.

SUGAR, LEMON, AND HONEY WAX

Creates a natural wax for hair removal.

Ingredients

- 1 cup sugar
- 1 tbsp lemon juice
- 1 tbsp honey

Instructions

- Combine the ingredients in a small saucepan and heat over medium heat. Stir occasionally until the mixture thickens into a wax-like consistency. Remove from the heat and allow to cool slightly, but ensure it is still warm enough to spread easily. Apply the mixture in the direction of hair growth, and place a fabric strip over it. Press firmly and then quickly pull the strip off against the direction of hair growth.

PAPAYA AND TURMERIC MASK

Exfoliates and reduces hair growth over time.

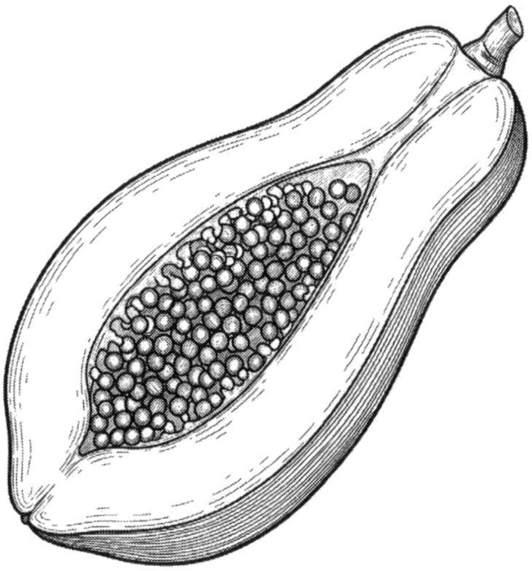

Ingredients

- half a cup mashed ripe papaya
- 1 tbsp turmeric powder

Instructions

- Mash the papaya in a bowl until it forms a smooth paste. Add the turmeric powder and mix well until combined. Apply the mask to areas with unwanted hair, massaging it in gently. Leave the mask on for about 20-30 minutes. Rinse off with warm water and repeat the treatment three times a week. Over time, the enzymes in papaya and the properties of turmeric may help slow down hair growth.

SUN PROTECTION: HERBAL REMEDIES TO SHIELD THE SKIN

Protect your skin from harmful UV rays with natural ingredients that not only shield but also soothe sun-exposed skin, keeping it healthy and radiant.

CARROT SEED OIL SUNSCREEN

Naturally protects the skin from sun damage.

Ingredients

- 2 tbsp carrot seed oil
- 4 tbsp coconut oil

Instructions

- Mix the carrot seed oil and coconut oil in a small bowl. Stir until fully combined. Apply the mixture to your skin 20 minutes before sun exposure, making sure to cover all areas you plan to expose to the sun. The sunscreen should be reapplied at two-hour intervals, or after swimming. This is a mild natural alternative and may not offer the same level of protection as commercial sunscreens.

ALOE VERA AND GREEN TEA AFTER-SUN SPRAY

Reduces inflammation and promotes healing.

Ingredients

- a quarter cup aloe vera gel
- a quarter cup cooled green tea

Instructions:

- Mix the fresh aloe vera gel and cooled green tea in a small spray bottle. Shake well to combine. Spritz generously onto sunburned or irritated skin for instant cooling and soothing relief. Use as often as needed for cooling relief, especially after sun exposure or when skin feels inflamed.

RASPBERRY SEED OIL LOTION

Offers mild sun protection and deep hydration.

Ingredients

- 2 tbsp raspberry seed oil
- 2 tbsp shea butter

Instructions

- Melt the shea butter in a double boiler or microwave until it becomes liquid. Once melted, add the raspberry seed oil and mix well. Let the mixture cool slightly before applying it to your skin as a lotion. Use especially after sun exposure for soothing and moisturizing benefits.

CHAPTER 14:

NATURAL CLEANING SOLUTIONS

Herbal and natural cleaning solutions offer a simple, eco-friendly way to keep your home clean while avoiding synthetic ingredients. By using common household items and the power of essential oils, you can create effective, non-toxic cleaners that are safe for both your family and the environment. These easy-to-make recipes provide a healthier, sustainable alternative to conventional cleaning products.

ALL-PURPOSE CLEANER: VERSATILE SOLUTION FOR MULTIPLE SURFACES

Tackle dirt and grime naturally with this all-purpose cleaner, perfect for a variety of surfaces and free from harsh chemicals. Give your hands a 10-minute soak, then pat them dry.

VINEGAR AND BAKING SODA SPRAY

Cleans countertops, sinks, and more.

Ingredients

- ½ cup white vinegar
- 2 tbsp baking soda
- 10 drops lemon essential oil (or tea tree oil)
- 2 cups water
- 1 spray bottle

Instructions

- In a large mixing cup, combine white vinegar and baking soda slowly (it will fizz). Once the fizzing subsides, add water and essential oil. Pour the mixture into a spray bottle and shake gently before each use. Spray onto surfaces and wipe clean with a cloth or sponge. Avoid using on marble, granite, or other natural stone surfaces, as vinegar can damage them.

GLASS AND MIRROR CLEANER: STREAK-FREE SHINE

Get a sparkling, streak-free finish on your glass and mirrors with this natural cleaner, leaving surfaces gleaming without any harsh chemicals.

VINEGAR AND WATER SOLUTION

Leaves glass surfaces streak-free and gleaming.

Ingredients

- ½ cup white vinegar
- ½ cup water
- 1 spray bottle

Instructions

- In a spray bottle, combine equal parts white vinegar and water. Shake well to mix. Spray onto glass and mirror surfaces. Wipe clean with a lint-free cloth or crumpled newspaper for a streak-free shine.

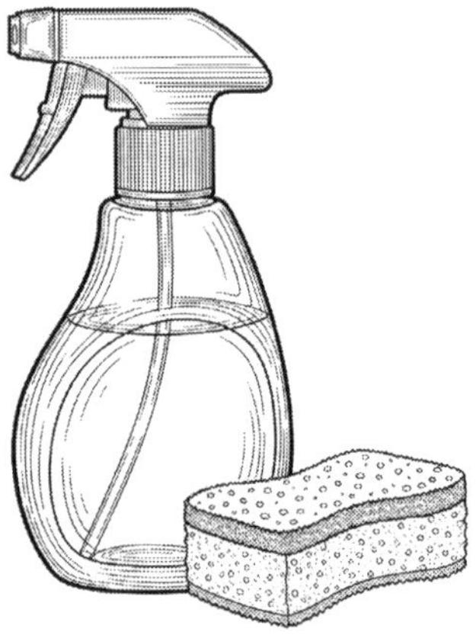

BATHROOM CLEANER: TACKLE SOAP SCUM AND MILDEW

Fight soap scum and mildew naturally with this powerful bathroom cleaner, using plant-based ingredients to keep your bathroom fresh, clean, and free from harsh chemicals.

BAKING SODA AND CASTILE SOAP PASTE

Cleans and removes buildup on bathroom surfaces.

Ingredients

- 1½ cups baking soda
- ½ cup liquid Castile soap
- a sponge

Instructions

- In a mixing bowl, combine baking soda and liquid Castile soap. Stir well to form a thick paste. Apply the paste to bathroom surfaces, such as sinks, tubs, and tiles. Scrub with a sponge to remove soap scum and mildew buildup. Rinse thoroughly with warm water to leave surfaces clean and fresh. For tough buildup, let the paste sit for 10–15 minutes before scrubbing.

FLOOR CLEANER: SAFE FOR VARIOUS FLOORING TYPES

Keep your floors spotless and safe with this gentle, natural cleaner, perfect for a variety of flooring types without the risk of damage or harsh chemicals.

VINEGAR AND WATER MOP SOLUTION

Cleans floors without leaving residue.

Ingredients

- 1 cup white vinegar
- 1 gallon warm water

Instructions

- Mix vinegar with warm water. Mop floors as usual, being careful not to over-wet wood surfaces.

AIR FRESHENER: NATURAL FRAGRANCE FOR YOUR HOME

Transform the air in your home with a refreshing, natural fragrance, using pure essential oils to create a clean, uplifting atmosphere without any artificial scents.

ESSENTIAL OIL SPRAY

Neutralizes odors and adds a pleasant fragrance.

Ingredients

- 1 cup water or vodka
- 10-20 drops of your favorite essential oil, or make a custom blend

Instructions:

- Fill a spray bottle with water or vodka. Add the essential oil (adjust based on fragrance strength preference). Shake well to combine and spritz around your home to freshen the air and neutralize odors. If you are using water as the base, shake the bottle before every use.

DISHWASHING LIQUID: GENTLE AND EFFECTIVE

This natural dish soap tackles grease with ease while being gentle on your hands.

CASTILE SOAP BLEND

Cuts grease without harsh chemicals.

Ingredients

- ½ cup warm distilled water
- 2 tsp kosher salt
- ½ cup white vinegar
- ½ cup Castile soap
- 1 tsp lemon juice

Instructions

- In a mixing bowl, combine distilled water and kosher salt. Stir until the salt dissolves. Add white vinegar, Castile soap, and lemon juice. Mix thoroughly until well combined. Pour the mixture into a bottle for easy use. Use this blend as you would commercial dish soap to clean dishes, remove grease, or wash surfaces.

LAUNDRY DETERGENTS: ECO-FRIENDLY FABRIC CARE

Keep your clothes fresh and clean with this natural, eco-friendly detergent that works hard on stains while being gentle on your fabrics.

BORAX AND WASHING SODA MIX

Cleans clothes effectively while being eco-friendly.

Ingredients

- 2 cups grated natural soap (e.g., Castile soap)
- 4 cups boiling water
- 2 cups washing soda
- 2 cups borax
- 30 cups warm water

Instructions

- In a large bucket, dissolve grated natural soap in some boiling water. Add washing soda and borax to the mixture. Stir until fully dissolved. Pour the remaining warm water in and mix well. Let the mixture sit overnight to thicken and set. Use up to half a cup of the mixture per load of laundry.

SOAP NUT LAUNDRY DETERGENT

Natural, eco-friendly laundry detergent suitable for sensitive skin.

Ingredients

- 10-15 soap nuts (saponin-rich fruit pods)
- 4 cups of water

Instructions

- Place the soap nuts into a muslin or cotton bag. In a saucepan, bring water to a boil and add the bag of soap nuts. Let the soap nuts simmer for 10-15 minutes to extract the saponin. Remove from the heat and allow the liquid to cool slightly. Strain the liquid into a container to separate the soap nuts from the liquid. Use about half a cup of the soap nut liquid for a normal load of laundry. Soap nuts can be reused up to three times. Simply dry them after each use and store them for the next batch. For extra fragrance, you can add a few drops of your favorite essential oil to the detergent.

DRAIN CLEANER: UNCLOG AND DEODORIZE NATURALLY

Keep your drains clear and smelling fresh with this easy, natural solution that tackles clogs and odors.

BAKING SODA AND VINEGAR FLUSH

Clears blockages and eliminates odors.

Ingredients

- ½ cup baking soda
- ¼ cup white vinegar
- boiling water (enough to flush the drain)

Instructions

Pour baking soda down the drain. Follow with white vinegar. You'll notice bubbling and fizzing as the ingredients react. Let the mixture sit for about 15 minutes to allow the reaction to break down any buildup. After 15 minutes, flush the drain with boiling water to clear any blockages and freshen the drain. Use this method monthly to keep your drains clean and smelling fresh!

PART THREE:

SAFE AND PRACTICAL PRACTICES

CHAPTER 15:

SAFETY AND DOSAGE GUIDE

Using herbal remedies safely starts with understanding proper dosing and precautions. Unlike prescription drugs, herbal medicines aren't strictly regulated, so users are urged to take all the steps needed to ensure their safety.

DOSAGE AND QUALITY

Herbal dosages vary based on age, weight, and health conditions. A dose suitable for a healthy adult may not be safe for a child or an elderly person. For example, echinacea, often used for immune support, should be taken short-term – no more than two weeks – to prevent overstimulating the immune system (John Hopkins Medicine, 2019). Herbs come in different forms, each requiring careful dosing:

- **Tinctures:** Highly concentrated, dosed in drops.
- **Teas:** Milder, requiring consistent consumption for effect.
- **Capsules and powders:** Standardized but still require careful adherence to recommended amounts.

Titration dosing is a careful way of adjusting the amount of an herbal supplement or remedy to find the right dose. It's generally one of the safest ways you can go about using natural treatments. You start with a small amount and gradually increase it until you feel the desired effect, while watching for any negative reactions. If you notice side effects, you lower the amount you take. This method is especially helpful for strong or new herbs and tinctures to reduce risks and increase benefits.

The quality of herbs affects both safety and effectiveness. Contaminants like heavy metals pose health risks, so it's essential to choose organic, high-quality sources. Reputable manufacturers test for purity, ensuring safety and efficacy (*Traditional Herbal Medicines,* 2008). Checking FDA alerts and researching herbs on PubMed or Google Scholar can help you make better choices. Keeping a health journal to note herbs, dosages, and side effects can make using herbs safer, especially when you discuss it with a healthcare provider.

A NOTE ON SIDE EFFECTS

Herbal remedies can cause mild to severe side effects. Common reactions include nausea or digestive issues, which may signal a need to adjust the dosage. For example, fenugreek, often used for menstrual cramps or milk production, can cause nausea, headaches, and dizziness (Hassen et al., 2022). More serious reactions, such as difficulty breathing or skin rashes, require immediate medical attention. But that's not the only risk. Some herbs interfere with medications, which can prove dangerous, such as:

- *St. John's Wort*, which can reduce birth control effectiveness (John Hopkins Medicine, 2019).
- *Ginkgo Biloba*, which may increase bleeding risk when combined with blood thinners.

More dangerously, kava and ephedra can harm the liver or increase the risk of heart attacks and strokes (Hassen et al., 2022). Therefore, it's always a good idea to stop any herbal treatments two weeks before you are scheduled for surgery. Additionally, it's important to inform your healthcare professional about the herbal remedies you have been using and for how long. This information is crucial for healthcare professionals to provide the appropriate medical treatment or intervention. Consulting a trained herbalist or healthcare provider ensures safe use, especially for those who fall into vulnerable groups such as:

- **Pregnant and nursing women:** Pregnant women need to be careful with herbs. While ginger can help with nausea, other herbs might cause issues like contractions, miscarriages, or early births. Fennel, for example, can change how drugs work in the body, possibly leading to unexpected results (Sarecka-Hujar and Szulc-Musioł, 2022).
- **People living with chronic illnesses:** Herbal use may worsen conditions or interfere with medications.
- **Children and the elderly:** Different metabolic responses require extra caution (John Hopkins Medicine, 2019).

Herbal medicine has many benefits, but safety is the most important thing. Following the right guidelines reduces risks and makes it more effective. Better regulations, clinical trials, and safety standards will help make sure that the benefits of herbal medicine are increased while risks are lowered. Until then, it's important to balance expert advice with your own caution when adding herbs to your health routine.

YOUR NEXT STEPS

Every leaf, root, and flower holds a story – one shaped by generations of healers, wisdom keepers, and everyday people who have trusted the gifts of the earth. By exploring this path, you're not just learning how to make teas, tinctures, and salves; you're stepping into an ancient dialogue between humans and nature, where listening is just as important as doing. The plants you've met along the way – chamomile for calm, echinacea for resilience, peppermint for renewal – are now part of your own healing journey. But this is only the beginning.

One of the most empowering aspects of herbalism is its ability to put wellness into your own hands. Whether you're tending to a minor ailment, strengthening your immune system, or simply deepening your connection with the natural world, each step you take strengthens your ability to care for yourself and those around you. But with this empowerment comes responsibility – responsibility to ensure safe practices, to honor the traditions that have carried this knowledge forward, and to respect the plants themselves by using them ethically and sustainably.

As you continue down this path, I encourage you to remain curious. Herbalism is a lifelong practice, and the learning never stops. Keep experimenting, keep questioning, and keep exploring new ways to integrate plant medicine into your life. Seek out books, courses, and communities that expand your knowledge. Grow your own herbs, support local herbalists, and look for sustainably sourced ingredients whenever possible. If you're drawn to a particular plant, spend time with it – observe it in nature, learn its history, and discover its many uses.

If this book has sparked your interest, there are so many ways to go deeper. Consider exploring resources like:

- *Rosemary Gladstar's Medicinal Herbs: A Beginner's Guide* – A fantastic introduction with easy-to-follow recipes and foundational knowledge.
- *The Herbal Medicine-Maker's Handbook* by James Green – A hands-on guide to making herbal preparations at home.
- *Medical Herbalism* by David Hoffmann – A more in-depth look at herbal therapeutics, plant chemistry, and traditional wisdom.
- *Herbal Antibiotics* & *Herbal Antivirals* by Stephen Harrod Buhner – Focused on using herbs for infections and immune support.
- *Braiding Sweetgrass* by Robin Wall Kimmerer – A poetic and insightful look at Indigenous plant wisdom and our relationship with nature.
- *The Medicinal Gardening Handbook* by Dede Cummings – Helps you grow your own healing plants.

Beyond books, there are apps and online communities that can enrich your experience with herbal remedies considerably. Consider keeping a personal journal to track your experiences.

Remember, your herbal journey is uniquely yours, shaped by your needs, environment, and intuition. Trust that process.

So, as you step forward, take this knowledge with you – not as a rigid set of rules, but as an invitation. An invitation to be more present, more connected, and more in tune with the rhythms of the natural world. Now, go forth and explore, create, and heal. The plants are waiting.

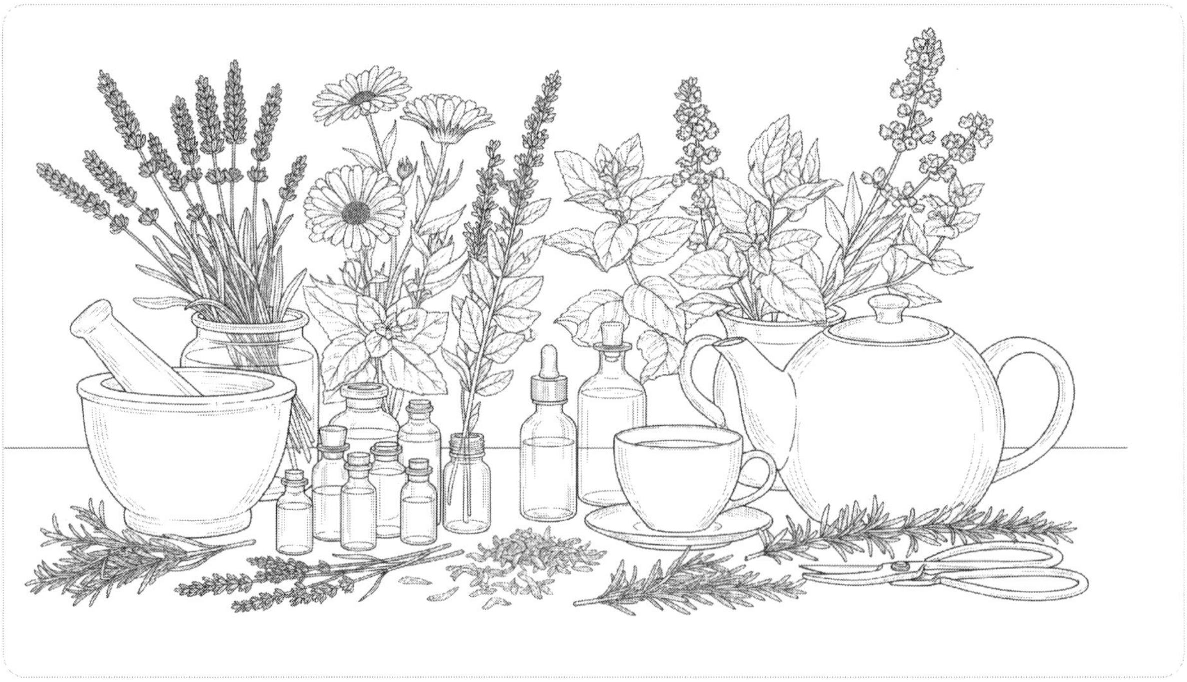

REFERENCES

- Ansary, J., Forbes-Hernández, T. Y., Gil, E., Cianciosi, D., Zhang, J., Elexpuru-Zabaleta, M., Simal-Gandara, J., Giampieri, F., & Battino, M. (2020). Potential Health Benefit of Garlic Based on Human Intervention Studies: A Brief Overview. *Antioxidants, 9*(7). https://doi.org/10.3390/antiox9070619
- Arreola, R., Quintero-Fabián, S., López-Roa, R. I., Flores-Gutiérrez, E. O., Reyes-Grajeda, J. P., Carrera-Quintanar, L., & Ortuño-Sahagún, D. (2015). Immunomodulation and Anti-Inflammatory Effects of Garlic Compounds. *Journal of Immunology Research, 2015*(401630), 1–13. https://doi.org/10.1155/2015/401630
- Ashpari, Z. (2024, September 30). *The Calming Effects of Passionflower*. Healthline. https://www.healthline.com/health/anxiety/calming-effects-of-passionflower
- *Ashwagandha: Is it helpful for stress, anxiety, or sleep?* (2023, October 24). Ods.od.nih.gov. https://ods.od.nih.gov/factsheets/Ashwagandha-HealthProfessional/
- Benzie, I. F. F., & Wachtel-Galor, S. (2011). *Herbal medicine: Biomolecular and clinical aspects* (2nd ed.). Crc Press, Cop.
- *Biodiversity and Wild Herbs - Sustainable Herbs Initiative*. (2021, November 4). Sustainable Herbs Initiative. https://sustainableherbsinitiative.org/explore/issues/sustainability/
- Boling, J. (2010, May 14). *33 herbal products you can make at home*. Everygreenherb.com; Janice Boling. https://www.everygreenherb.com/lotionsPotions.html?srsltid=AfmBOopHbBoHsWhn90Ptg17ebjA17CJZQuunhuDXti4MzKJjuTdDcZHX
- Bowman, J. (2023, October 30). *The Many Benefits of Lavender for Mood, Sleep, Hair, and Skin*. Healthline; Healthline Media. https://www.healthline.com/health/what-lavender-can-do-for-you
- Bowman, R., Taylor, J., Muggleton, S., & Davis, D. (2021). Biophysical effects, safety and efficacy of raspberry leaf use in pregnancy: a systematic integrative review. *BMC Complementary Medicine and Therapies, 21*(1). https://doi.org/10.1186/s12906-021-03230-4
- Braveman, J. (2024, April 16). *Fennel: Health Benefits, Nutrients, and Recipes*. WebMD. https://www.webmd.com/food-recipes/health-benefits-fennel
- Calhoun, L. (2024, June). Essential Tools for Your Home Apothecary. *Calhoun Farm*. https://calhounfarmstead.com/blogs/news/essential-tools-for-your-home-apothecary
- Carson, C. F., Hammer, K. A., & Riley, T. V. (2006). Melaleuca alternifolia (Tea Tree) Oil: a Review of Antimicrobial and Other Medicinal Properties. *Clinical Microbiology Reviews, 19*(1), 50–62. https://doi.org/10.1128/cmr.19.1.50-62.2006
- Coleman, A. (2023, January 9). "*Poaching can lead to local succulent species becoming extinct*." Farmer's Weekly. https://www.farmersweekly.co.za/agri-news/south-africa/poaching-can-lead-to-local-succulent-species-becoming-extinct/
- Dietrich-Marsh, J. (2020, May 26). *What's in my medicine cabinet? (a natural doctor and mom of four)*. All Natural Family Doc. https://allnaturalfamilydoc.com/medicine-cabinet/
- Easley, T., & Horne, S. H. (2016). *The modern herbal dispensatory: a medicine-making guide*. North Atlantic Books.
- *Echinacea*. (2020, July). NCCIH. https://www.nccih.nih.gov/health/echinacea

- *Elderberry.* (2025). Rochester.edu. https://www.urmc.rochester.edu/encyclopedia/content?contenttypeid=19&contentid=elderberry
- Elendu, C. (2024, July 12). The evolution of ancient healing practices: From shamanism to Hippocratic medicine: A review. *Medicine.* https://doi.org/10.1097/MD.0000000000039005
- *Evidence-Based Facts for What You Put On Your Face.* (2022, September 1). Healthline. https://www.healthline.com/health/beauty-skin-care/skin-care-ingredients-dictionary
- Frobese, J. (2021). *Growing and preserving my own herbs (food preservation forum at permies).* Permies.com. https://permies.com/t/152559/Growing-preserving-herbs
- *German chamomile.* (n.d.). Mount Sinai Health System. https://www.mountsinai.org/health-library/herb/german-chamomile
- Gill, H. B. (1972). *The apothecary in colonial Virginia.* Williamsburg, Va., Colonial Williamsburg Foundation; Distributed By The University Press Of Virginia, Charlottesville, Va.
- Hammoudi Halat, D., Krayem, M., Khaled, S., & Younes, S. (2022). A Focused Insight into Thyme: Biological, Chemical, and Therapeutic Properties of an Indigenous Mediterranean Herb. *Nutrients, 14*(10), 2104. https://doi.org/10.3390/nu14102104
- Hassen, G., Belete, G., Carrera, K. G., Iriowen, R. O., Araya, H., Alemu, T., Solomon, N., Bam, D. S., Nicola, S. M., Araya, M. E., Debele, T., Zouetr, M., and Jain, N. (2022, July 15). Clinical Implications of Herbal Supplements in Conventional Medical Practice: A US Perspective. *Cureus.* https://doi.org/10.7759/cureus.26893
- Heron, B. (2023, January 25). *How to make a herbal salve.* Earthsong Seeds. https://earthsongseeds.co.uk/recipes/how-to-make-a-herbal-salve/
- *How to Harvest and Dry Herbs for Storage.* (2016, July 13). Grow a Good Life. https://growagoodlife.com/harvest-dry-herbs/
- How to Make Herbal Salves. (2025). *Learningherbs.com.* https://www.learningherbs.com/blog/how-to-make-herbal-salves
- Jessicka. (n.d.). Organizing Your Home Apothecary. *Blog.mountainroseherbs.com.* https://blog.mountainroseherbs.com/apothecary-storage
- John Hopkins Medicine. (2019). *Herbal medicine.* John Hopkins Medicine. https://www.hopkinsmedicine.org/health/wellness-and-prevention/herbal-medicine
- Kennedy, D. O., Bonnländer, B., Lang, S. C., Pischel, I., Forster, J., Khan, J., Jackson, P. A., & Wightman, E. L. (2020). Acute and Chronic Effects of Green Oat (Avena sativa) Extract on Cognitive Function and Mood during a Laboratory Stressor in Healthy Adults: A Randomised, Double-Blind, Placebo-Controlled Study in Healthy Humans. *Nutrients, 12*(6), 1598. https://doi.org/10.3390/nu12061598
- Kovacevic, M. (2024). *Seeds of Sisterhood.* Thorpe-Bowker.
- Leslie, H. A., J. M. van Velzen, M., Brandsma, S. H., Vethaak, D., Garcia-Vallejo, J. J., & Lamoree, M. H. (2022). Discovery and quantification of plastic particle pollution in human blood. *Environment International, 163*(107199), 107199. https://doi.org/10.1016/j.envint.2022.107199
- Lieberman, C. (2023, April 12). 10 Benefits of Herbal Medicine. *Wild Abundance.* https://www.wildabundance.net/blog/10-benefits-of-herbal-medicine/
- Ling, S. (2024, October). *Drying Herbs: The Easiest Way to Preserve Your Harvest.* Bricks 'N Blooms with Stacy Ling. https://stacyling.com/drying-herbs-the-easy-way/
- Mason. (n.d.). Must-Have Tools for Herbalists. *Blog.mountainroseherbs.com.* https://blog.mountainroseherbs.com/tools-for-herbalists
- Meixner, M. (2024, November 26). *Astragalus: An Ancient Root With Health Benefits.* Healthline; Healthline Media. https://www.healthline.com/nutrition/astragalus
- Modi, M., & Modi, K. (2021). *Ginger Root.* PubMed; StatPearls Publishing. https://www.ncbi.nlm.nih.gov/books/NBK565886/
- Pan, S.-Y., Litscher, G., Gao, S.-H., Zhou, S.-F., Yu, Z.-L., Chen, H.-Q., Zhang, S.-F., Tang, M.-K., Sun, J.-N., & Ko, K.-M. (2014). Historical Perspective of Traditional Indigenous Medical Practices: The Current Renaissance and Conservation of Herbal Resources. *Evidence-Based Complementary and Alternative Medicine, 2014*(525340), 1–20. https://doi.org/10.1155/2014/525340
- *Peppermint.* (n.d.). Mount Sinai Health System. https://www.mountsinai.org/health-library/herb/peppermint
- Pereira, C. G., Barreira, L., Bijttebier, S., Pieters, L., Marques, C., Santos, T. F., Rodrigues, M. J., Varela, J., and Custódio, L. (2018, March 16). Health promoting potential of herbal teas and tinctures from Artemisia campestris subsp. maritima: from traditional remedies to prospective products. *Scientific Reports.* https://doi.org/10.1038/s41598-018-23038-6

- Remedies, N. Y. (2023, March 13). Using herbs: Teas versus tinctures. *Neal's Yard Remedies; Neal's Yard Remedies*. https://www.nealsyardremedies.com/blogs/wellbeing/using-herbs-teas-versus-tinctures
- Saras. (2025). *Natural Remedies for People*. Sarassuperbherbs.com. https://www.sarassuperbherbs.com/page/Natural-Remedies-for-People
- Sarecka-Hujar, B., and Szulc-Musioł, B. (2022, January 12). Herbal Medicines – Are They Effective and Safe during Pregnancy? *Pharmaceutics*. https://doi.org/10.3390/pharmaceutics14010171
- Shenefelt, P. D. (2011). *Herbal Treatment for Dermatologic Disorders* (I. F. F. Benzie and S. Wachtel-Galor, Eds.). PubMed; CRC Press/Taylor and Francis. https://www.ncbi.nlm.nih.gov/books/NBK92761/
- Thomas, C. (2023, February 15). *Herbal Tinctures - How to Make Your Own*. Homesteading Family. https://homesteadingfamily.com/herbal-tinctures-how-to-make-your-own/
- Traditional Herbal Medicines: a Guide to Their Safer Use. (2008, September). *British Journal of Clinical Pharmacology*. https://doi.org/10.1111/j.1365-2125.2008.03259.x
- *Traditional medicine*. (2023). World Health Organization. https://www.who.int/news-room/questions-and-answers/item/traditional-medicine
- Turker, A. U., & Gurel, E. (2005). Common mullein (Verbascum thapsus L.): recent advances in research. *Phytotherapy Research, 19*(9), 733–739. https://doi.org/10.1002/ptr.1653
- *Valerian*. (2020, October). NCCIH. https://www.nccih.nih.gov/health/valerian
- Wallace, T. C. (2019). Health Effects of Coconut Oil-A Narrative Review of Current Evidence. *Journal of the American College of Nutrition, 38*(2), 97–107. https://doi.org/10.1080/07315724.2018.1497562
- White, A. (2019, August 7). *Why You Should Grow Your Own Medicine Cabinet* | Iowa Herbalist. Adrian White | Jupiter Ridge Farm. https://iowaherbalist.com/2019/08/07/farmer-herbalist-why-you-should-grow-your-own-indoor-medicine-cabinet/
- Whitlock, C. (2020). *Botanicum medicinale: a modern herbal of medicinal plants*. The Mit Press.
- Wilt, A. (2024, November 20). *65 Inspiring Quotes About Nature*. Southern Living. https://www.southernliving.com/culture/nature-quotes
- Wust, M. (2017, October 13). The Evolution of the Apothecary for the Apothe-curious – PR News. *Pennmedicine.org*. https://www.pennmedicine.org/news/news-blog/2017/october/the-evolution-of-the-apothecary-for-the-apothecurious
- Zimmermann, L., Bartosova, Z., Braun, K., Oehlmann, J., Völker, C., & Wagner, M. (2021). Plastic Products Leach Chemicals That Induce In Vitro Toxicity under Realistic Use Conditions. *Environmental Science & Technology, 55*(17), 11814–11823. https://doi.org/10.1021/acs.est.1c01103

FROM THE AUTHOR

Thank you for making it this far!

I greatly appreciate the time you took to give my book a read.

As a passionate advocate of natural health and an independent writer, your attention means a lot and I hope I am making a difference in your home herbalism journey.

If you have 60 seconds, it would mean the world to me to hear your honest feedback on Amazon. It does wonders for the book and I love hearing about your experience!

To leave your feedback:

- Open your camera app
- Point your mobile device at the QR code below
- The review page will appear in your web browser on your device

Thank you!

James J Cork

Made in the USA
Monee, IL
11 November 2026

2b5cc5ae-c263-4b03-9fa1-c852e3410936R02